The
Microbiome
Connection

The
Microbiome
Connection

Your Guide to IBS, SIBO, and Low-Fermentation Eating

DR. MARK PIMENTEL & DR. ALI REZAIE

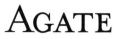

GOODL/FE
low fermentation eating

www.thegoodlfe.com

Agate trade paperback printing: March 2024

Printed in the United States

10 9 8 7 6 5 4 3 2 1   24 25 26 27 28

ISBN-13: 978-1-57284-334-9
ISBN-10: 1-57284-334-9
eISBN-13: 978-1-57284-863-4
eISBN-10: 1-57284-863-4

Library of Congress Cataloging-in-Publication Data is available from the Library of Congress

Surrey is an imprint of Agate Publishing. Agate books are available in bulk at discount prices. For more information, visit Agatepublishing.com.

Produced by Exquisite Corp.
exqcorp.com

Contents

We dedicate this book to all with a chronic invisible illness:
to those who suffer but don't look sick; to those who hurt but routine
tests are inconclusive; to those who agonize in silence. There is only
one roadmap forward: knowledge and awareness!

Introduction to IBS, SIBO, and Their Overlap

I f you come away with only one notion from this book, let it be optimism! If you have Irritable Bowel Syndrome (IBS), you are not alone, and you can get better. And if you are among the millions of people who have Small Intestinal Bacterial Overgrowth (SIBO), a debilitating condition that occurs when bacteria that normally grow in other parts of the gut begin to grow in the small intestine, we share our expertise along with a unique SIBO diet and treatment plan to help ease your symptoms. We know . . . it's already confusing. Are IBS and SIBO the same thing or are they different conditions? Can SIBO occur without IBS? We'll guide you through the answers to these questions as you read this book.

IBS

The most common gastrointestinal (GI) condition in the United States is IBS, which is characterized by abdominal pain/discomfort, bloating, and altered bowel habits (diarrhea or constipation or both). IBS affects millions of people of all ages, and it appears to be slightly more common among women than men. Economically and socially, the cost of IBS can be significant, as those coping with IBS often miss days of work or school.

Many people who suffer from chronic IBS choose not to travel on planes, trains, and buses, and avoid dates or outings with family or friends for fear of having to explain their bathroom trips and their pain and discomfort. After all, talking about your bowel movements or how bloated you feel is not considered polite conversation in most circles. So the people you spend time with may never know about your struggle.

As IBS becomes a better-recognized disease, it will be easier to discuss. You can and should talk about IBS to your health-care providers, family, and friends. We know so much more about IBS, and we continue to learn more every year. The more you know about IBS, the better equipped you are to talk about it, and the less its burden becomes. By educating your family and friends, you can both broaden support and lessen the stigma of IBS.

Primary care doctors and health-care personnel must keep up with so many illnesses, so it's important that we educate them about new IBS information. The more doctors—not just gastroenterologists, but all health-care providers—know about it, the better off IBS patients will be. As physically challenging as it may be, IBS gut pain can be alleviated with proper diagnosis and treatment. Yet we often see patients suffer as they bounce between Western medicine and alternative medicine, getting differing opinions and advice from physicians, dietitians, nurse practitioners, and naturopaths. In some situations, the advice or treatment may worsen their symptoms.

What's Wrong with Me?

The primary problem is that no one answers the ultimate question: What's wrong with me? Patients tell us, "All I hear is what I don't have. All my tests are negative. Are there no tests to confirm my illness?" or "I don't know what's wrong with me; I'm starting to believe it's all in my head." And when you don't know what's going on, you may be given procedures, tests, or treatments that are potentially harmful.

IBS is not a fatal illness. It won't lead to cancer. It hasn't yet killed anyone, the way heart disease or kidney disease can. But let's be clear . . . just because IBS isn't lethal, doesn't mean it's not a problem. It's not a lifestyle condition wherein patients are simply worried about what they eat. Moreover, IBS suffering is intense, as we'll discuss later. In fact, some studies have shown that people with IBS have a lower quality of life than people with heart disease. The other problem with the notion that "IBS is not a deadly disease" is that there's less effort to fund research, and therefore our scientific understanding of IBS has been slow to evolve.

IBS Prevalence

IBS is extremely common. If you're reading this book on a bus or train right now, look around you: one in seven of your fellow passengers likely has IBS. Just 10 years ago, people with IBS often felt socially isolated; their symptoms were dismissed by family and friends as being imaginary, and there was little hope that the symptoms would ever disappear, or at least lessen and improve. This is not the case today. Over the last 15 years, research into IBS, gut motility, the gut's immune system, and the vast inner workings of the gut's microbiome (the trillions of bacteria, fungi, and viruses harbored in the gut) has been groundbreaking. Our work as clinicians and researchers has convinced us that IBS patients can experience an improved quality of life, engage successfully at work, and lead full, active lives. Many, if not most, IBS patients can find partial or complete relief from this often-debilitating disease.

Is IBS a Disease?

Notice that we just referred to IBS as a "disease." Doesn't IBS stand for irritable bowel "syndrome"? As you read through the chapters of this book you'll see that IBS *is* a legitimate "disease" and that the word "syndrome" may no longer apply. In fact, we believe there's hope for a course of action and an IBS-free future. We look forward to a time when IBS is no longer a chronic disease, but a manageable, finite illness that disappears with proper diagnosis and treatment. In this book, we share what we have learned and how we are now treating IBS. Most importantly, we show you how to empower yourself and lead a normal life again—a life, we hope, that is entirely absent of IBS or IBS symptoms.

The SIBO Subgroup

We also wrote this book to increase awareness and understanding among the subgroup of IBS patients who have SIBO. Through our research, we have found that about three-quarters of patients—as many as 30 million Americans—who have met the diagnostic criteria for IBS have taken a breath test that suggests they have SIBO. We hope this book will pave the way to more SIBO research and funding to improve the treatment of this large community. So how do SIBO and IBS intertwine?

Research on the effects of the microbiome on IBS/SIBO was in its infancy when Mark Pimentel, MD, wrote his first book—A New IBS Solution—more than 10 years ago. Since then there have been many new discoveries about the bacterial composition of the small intestine, the autoimmune cause of SIBO, and the treatment for SIBO.

Selected Treatment Options

When Dr. Mark Pimentel's book was published, there were few treatment options for IBS or SIBO; in fact, 10 years ago there were only a few drugs approved by the Food and Drug Administration (FDA) to treat IBS. Today there are eight drugs for IBS on the market: five drugs to treat IBS with constipation and three drugs to treat IBS with diarrhea. Importantly, none of these drugs are antidepressants or antipsychotics that are designed to relieve the stress that may be associated with IBS, but is not the cause of IBS. One drug, the antibiotic rifaximin, can eliminate or lessen bacteria in the gut. The other drugs alter motility to help move the bowels or to move fluid through the bowels to relieve the constipating symptoms of IBS. With the FDA now on board, pharmacological treatment of IBS is changing dramatically.

Dietary changes to treat IBS/SIBO have also evolved. Twenty years ago, you may have been advised not to eat any fiber or legumes, or to avoid foods that you found through personal experience didn't agree with you. Then the gluten-free and low-FODMAP diets were introduced. FOD-MAP is an acronym for "Fermentable Oligo-, Di-, Monosaccharides And Polyols." These are short-chain carbohydrates that are poorly absorbed in the small intestine, including wheat and beans. Studies have shown strong links between FODMAPs and the digestive symptoms of IBS/SIBO, including gas, bloating, stomach pain, diarrhea, and constipation.

Certain foods are linked to symptoms of IBS and SIBO, but it's not that simple. Multiple studies have shown that low-FODMAP diets can provide benefits for some people with these digestive symptoms. If you have IBS, chances are you've heard about the low-FODMAP diet. However, you can't be on a low-FODMAP diet forever. In its most restrictive form, adhering to this diet for three months or more can lead to macronutrient and micronutrient deficiencies (as shown by Dr. William Chey, Ann Arbor, Michigan). Over the last few years, researchers have shown that IBS/SIBO patients can eat a low-FODMAP diet, but must reintroduce the foods that were eliminated within four weeks to prevent nutrient deficiencies.

As outlined above, IBS and SIBO *are* related, and SIBO may be an important cause of IBS symptoms. In fact, IBS can indeed be SIBO- and microbiome-induced. In this book, we will focus on SIBO, as we have made the biggest leap in understanding the diagnosis and treatment for the SIBO group of IBS patients as compared to those without SIBO. We know the underlying medical cause of SIBO, how to diagnose it—whether it derives from a motility problem or from an imbalance of microbes in the gut—and the role of autoimmunity for those suffering from IBS. We know how to treat SIBO with antibiotics, followed by promotility drugs to help the bowels move and keep the microbiome balanced. SIBO is the most well-defined part of IBS, and we are making significant headway in its treatment.

SIBO Patients, Family Members, and Professionals

This book is not just for patients with IBS and SIBO; it can also be a learning tool for a family member of someone with SIBO to understand the daily struggles with these conditions. Physicians may also use this book to study the principles of how we understand IBS as a microbiome disease and to learn about the tools to handle patients with this aspect of IBS.

If you're a patient with SIBO, we hope this book will help you understand what's going on with your body. If you don't respond to treatment, you will know why your symptoms are sometimes unpredictable. You will be better able to manage your symptoms to achieve freedom from IBS and SIBO and you will also be better equipped to interact with your health-care professionals when they recommend a certain treatment or diet for you.

If you're the family member of a SIBO patient, you'll better understand why it's difficult for someone with this disorder to be comfortable at dinner because of food sensitivities or symptoms. You'll develop more understanding of the workings of a SIBO patient's body, which will lead to more empathy for your family member.

If you're a health-care professional, this book will help you better understand SIBO. Today's medical precepts change so quickly that you may not be aware of how many of your patients have been diagnosed with SIBO. This book will help you address the SIBO portion of concomitant medical problems.

If you're a dietitian, you may not be an expert in gastrointestinal diseases. The majority of dietitians help their patients with the nutritional aspects of diabetes, high blood pressure, and heart disease, but not necessarily IBS. Some dietitians only treat celiac disease or inflammatory bowel disease. This book can aid your understanding of what the IBS/SIBO patient needs in terms of diet as well as what has the potential to harm them.

We know of no other book that covers the entire spectrum of SIBO. This book provides simple explanations of what happens to IBS/SIBO patients from diagnosis to the end of treatment. We reveal changes that can occur in the body in terms of the underlying physical processes and symptoms that may develop. We also cite evidence-based management and treatment with both drugs and dietary changes.

Collectively, we have published hundreds of peer-reviewed journal articles on the topics in this book. Here we have transformed our research into a language that we hope is relatable and easy for you to understand. What's more, the book includes diagrams of how food travels through the digestive system and how bacteria are distributed throughout the gut, as well as a *meal plan guide* that includes which foods to eat in moderation and which foods to avoid because they will feed bacteria in the gut and potentially lead to more symptoms. We also provide *sample menus for breakfast, lunch, and dinner.*

You'll also learn about *the three pillars of SIBO management* to reduce problem bacteria, ideas to reduce symptoms, and *an elemental diet to starve out the non-beneficial bugs.* Finally, we *bust the 10 myths of IBS.*

What's Next?

We know of no other researchers who have studied IBS/SIBO as intently as we have over the past 20 years. We have observed a sea change in how to think about these digestive disorders, and we hope this evolution continues. We now have significantly better understanding of gut motility and the microbiome as they relate to IBS/SIBO. And we look forward to the development of better IBS drugs and interventions that can affect the microbiome in ways that benefit you.

Bugs as Drugs and Drugs for Bugs

Because IBS and SIBO may be a microbiome disease, it is important to explain how practitioners and/or patients can use bugs as drugs. Examples include probiotics and other live microorganisms intended to normalize the microbiome. A lesser used treatment, known as fecal transplantation, involves an infusion of stool (feces) from a donor to treat IBS/SIBO that is refractory to other treatments.

We hope that by following the instructions this book provides, you can achieve the same positive changes we see every day in our IBS and SIBO patients.

CHAPTER 1

IBS and You

"I developed irritable bowel syndrome (IBS) last year after getting sick on vacation. Now I've gained 15 pounds. How can that be when I have diarrhea?"

"My family doesn't seem to get it. I can't eat that because I know I will be in pain and bloated. And still every day they try to encourage me to eat everything."

"I'm bloated. I'm full. I'm gaining weight. I'm fatigued. I feel foggy in the head after eating. My doctor told me I'll just have to learn to live with it."

"My belly is flat in the morning, but by the evening it looks like I am 6 months pregnant!"

These are just a few of the complaints and concerns we often hear from our IBS patients. Equally disheartening is the lack of compassion, the insufficient information, and the endless unhelpful solutions and suggestions they have been given before coming to see us: "The tests didn't show anything." "Try this prebiotic." "Try this probiotic." "You're allergic to gluten." "Relax and you'll get better." "You're drinking too much coffee." "You're not exercising enough." Sound familiar?

As practicing gastroenterologists and longtime IBS researchers, we're a group of IBS specialists who have published many journal articles and advocated for patients for decades. We have a connection and a commitment to our thousands of patients and to those of you dealing with IBS. We know quite well what you're going through and what you've been dealing with. We know now that IBS affects people both physically and psychologically. We've seen first-hand how IBS adversely affects both the family life and the professional life of our patients.

Before getting into the science of your gut and its microbiome, the small intestinal bacterial overgrowth (SIBO) in those of you afflicted with IBS, and all the different ways we have dealt with this disease, let's talk about the impact of IBS, its symptoms, its history, and the issues surrounding it.

IBS by the Numbers

The first step in understanding the impact of IBS is to comprehend how common it is. Globally, about 11 percent of the world has IBS. That's nearly 1 billion people. In the United States, an estimated 10 to 15 percent of the population has IBS (Figure 1.1). It's the most common gastrointestinal disorder and one of the most treated disorders encountered by physicians. There are nearly 4 million doctor visits per year for IBS in the US alone, meaning that it accounts for up to 12 percent of total visits to primary care doctors. IBS can start at any age, but most commonly occurs in people between the ages of 20 to 40, and it afflicts more women than men—60 to 65 percent of IBS sufferers are women.

Economically, IBS costs American society more than $21 billion a year in lost productivity at work and in medical expenses, with 13 percent of IBS patients missing at least one day of work or school per month due to their symptoms. (In comparison, building a two-way road from Seattle to Miami would cost $10 billion.) Because IBS is not a fatal illness and is not given priority in research funding despite the high costs to society, the National Institutes of Health allots only $5 million per year in research funding for IBS. Of the 45 million IBS sufferers, that amounts to 8 cents per IBS patient. That's not even enough to build two miles of that two-way road between Seattle and Miami!

Defining—and Redefining—IBS

Ever since it was coined in the 1950s, the term IBS has been known by a variety of names: irritable colon, spastic colon, nervous colon, spastic colitis, mucous colitis, spastic bowel, and recently "leaky gut." None of these names really describes the exact nature of IBS. As one example, all the names centered around the colon miss the mark. Even more confusing, terms like "colitis" are entirely misleading. Inflammation of the colon—the definition of colitis—is not present in IBS. We now know that IBS encompasses the entire digestive system, including the small intestine. It's not just about your colon.

IBS didn't have an official name until the 1970s. Having a stable name is important to prevent confusion, and it gives both the patients and the medical community common ground. Furthermore, "Irritable Bowel Syndrome" misrepresents the severity of the disease. Can you imagine being called "irritable," "bowel," and "syndrome"? Calling it a "syndrome" implies that it's not even a disease. "Syndrome" also leans on the now-dispelled belief that IBS is a disease of psychological origin.

Figure 1.1 IBS prevalence in perspective.

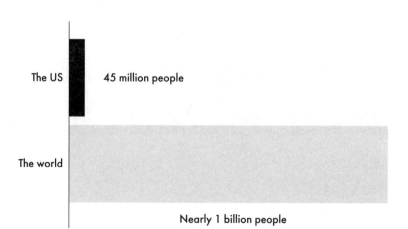

The US — 45 million people

The world — Nearly 1 billion people

In a sense, IBS wasn't just a disease without an agreed-upon name (that didn't officially occur until 1974); it was a disease without firm defining criteria. The cloud of doubt and uncertainty that has lurked around IBS for decades has only recently begun to lift. In 1988 a group of doctors—mostly gastroenterologists—released the first consensus-based set of standards used to diagnose IBS, known as the Rome Criteria. These standards were the result of 20 years of hard-fought efforts to redirect the growing field of research into gastrointestinal disorders. See Figure 1.2.

The main problem with the Rome Criteria is that they never really diagnosed IBS, as the criteria required first eliminating other diseases. For example, 70 to 80 percent of people with Crohn's disease meet the Rome Criteria, making the Rome Criteria useful only after the clinician eliminates other diseases (Figure 1.3). This concept is called a "diagnosis of exclusion," which we'll discuss later. In 1998, the updated Rome II Criteria were released. And in 1999, the connection between IBS and SIBO was officially established.

Figure 1.2 Evolution of IBS definitions over the years.

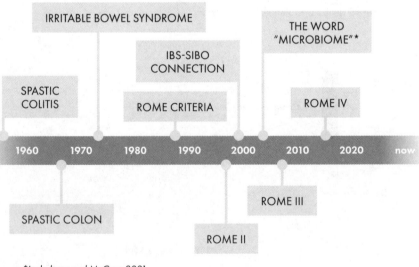

*Lederberg and McCray 2001

Figure 1.3 Overlap between Crohn's disease and Rome Criteria.

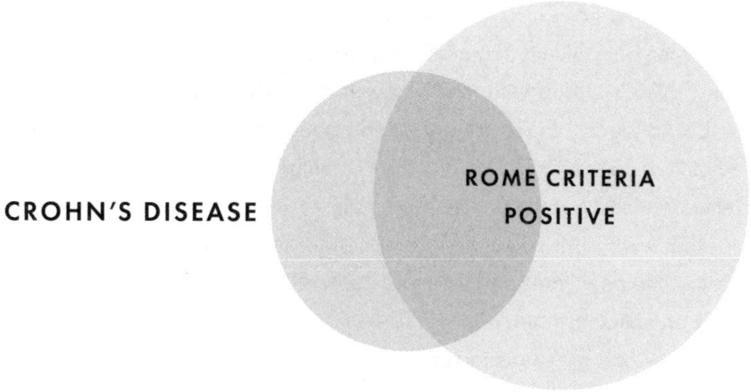

CROHN'S DISEASE

ROME CRITERIA
POSITIVE

Despite the above occurrences, the belief that IBS is a psychological condition, not a physical disease, persisted. In 1994, IBS was still listed in the fourth edition of the so-called bible of the psychiatric community, the *Diagnostic and Statistical Manual of Mental Disorders (DSM-IV)*. The DSM-IV wasn't updated until 2000. Ironically, the persistence that IBS was all in one's head led some IBS patients to be treated—with some success—using antipsychotics and antidepressants. Most of those treatments are less prescribed today.

In 2008, after a third meeting, the Rome III Criteria were released. Later in 2016, the Rome IV Criteria were released. In Rome IV, abdominal discomfort was removed from the definition of IBS and only abdominal pain was included in the criteria. Essentially, if you have persistent, weekly abdominal pain for more than three months that's associated with a change in bowel habits, you fit the diagnosis of IBS. No diagnostic testing or biomarkers have yet been incorporated into the Rome definition.

Why did experts quibble over the term abdominal discomfort versus abdominal pain? What does this have to do with you and what you're going through? Having better information allows your general practitioner or gastroenterologist to use more exact criteria when making a diagnosis of IBS. This means you can receive better care, have fewer diagnostic tests, and get back on the road to health more quickly. The data to support the modern Rome Criteria may diagnose IBS accurately, but the diagnosis is often based on comparison to healthy people with no symptoms. Also, the odds are you have IBS because it's much more common.

When our patients come to us, they don't say, "I have IBS." Instead, they ask, "What's wrong with me?" They don't really care about what the "S" in IBS stands for, or the latest agreed-upon name—they just want to know what their disease might be and they want the symptoms to stop. They want relief and they want to be healthy again.

That's why our focus and compassion are on our patients. The more precise the definitions and the more consistent the criteria for IBS, the better we can communicate with our patients and fellow physicians, and the faster we can make a diagnosis and start patients on a path to healing. Understandably, flip-flops over language and wording—for example, whether bloating or no bloating is a secondary or primary criteria—have led to confusion among patients and a lack of confidence among physicians. In fact, during a working group meeting of experts, more than three-quarters of physicians did not feel that the Rome III Criteria adequately reflected IBS in their practice or in their country. That's telling and that's a problem.

What Exactly Is IBS?

If you've had the following symptoms for three or more months, you have IBS: abdominal pain and/or discomfort, diarrhea, constipation, bloating, gas, urgency, incomplete evacuation, relief or worsening of pain with defecation, brain fog, early satiety (a sense of fullness without having eaten much), or both diarrhea and constipation. The last symptoms, diarrhea and constipation, may strike you as impossible, but they have now been classified as one of the three distinct types of IBS.

Types of IBS

First, there is *IBS-C*, meaning IBS with constipation. This type is found in 35 percent of patients. Second, there is *IBS-D*, which is IBS with diarrhea, found in 40 percent of patients. Third is *IBS-M* (mixed type), which is IBS with alternating bouts of diarrhea and constipation, found in 23 percent of patients. In this category, many patients don't know whether they will be hit with diarrhea or constipation. During the course of one day, they might be constipated in the morning, but have diarrhea in the afternoon. And within one bowel movement, their stool may be hard at the beginning and watery at the end. So, we now consider IBS-D and IBS-M as one type of IBS disease— Non-constipation IBS—and IBS-C is possibly a different disease, Constipation IBS.

Despite these categories of definition, if your complaint is diarrhea, how do you know for sure you don't have Crohn's disease, ulcerative colitis, or celiac disease? This is a problem. The existing criteria are so vague that doctors are not always sure. You may have test after test until your doctor rules out other GI diseases. Until now, there's not been a test to say "you have IBS and you don't need any other tests." There is now a definitive test that we'll discuss later in the book.

What IBS Is Not

We have advanced our understanding of IBS over the past 15 years, yet as recently as the 1970s, many doctors—including gastroenterologists— regarded IBS not as a disease but as a mental disorder, something that was purely psychological. For decades, most patients were told "It's all in your head" by their physicians. IBS wasn't real, it was psychosomatic, or if not all in your head, then it was your mental state that brought on the physical symptoms of IBS, including diarrhea, abdominal pain, and constipation.

The notion that stress can lead to IBS symptoms is one reason so many IBS patients have felt stigmatized and ostracized, and even doctors who argued against the psychosomatic causes of IBS were sidelined.

Until recently, doctors embraced this mind-over-body diagnosis in part because there was no concrete test for IBS. In fact, the most common path to an IBS diagnosis has been a diagnosis of exclusion: a doctor diagnosed IBS only after ruling out a long list of other potential causes that produced similar symptoms. Once again, the long list of alternate possibilities often included lactose intolerance, parasites, microscopic colitis, celiac disease, ulcerative colitis, and Crohn's disease. If after an exhaustive series of tests and procedures you did not fit squarely into the parameters of those other disorders, by process of elimination the doctor would diagnose IBS.

IBS is not like a broken leg or a rash. You can see a rash. You can see the break on an x-ray. Also, when you break your leg, you probably know how it happened—you fell on the ski slope. This leads to a specific type of care—a cast on your leg.

The cause of IBS is usually not so obvious, or commonly there are multiple causes. To complicate matters, the severity of the symptoms can vary and some patients experience both constipation and diarrhea. There is still confusion among doctors as to how to assess, and—more importantly—how to treat the combination of these two symptoms. Given the confusion about the causes and symptoms of IBS, it's not surprising that many of our patients come to us, having searched the internet, believing that the answer to their problems is probiotics or colonics or fecal transplantation!

A recent study found that 79 percent of community clinicians diagnosed IBS via exclusion, which resulted in more tests for their patients and significantly raised the direct costs of patient care. The extra testing (stool tests, colonoscopies, upper endoscopies, computed tomography scans, ultrasounds, and x-rays) and the recommended surgeries (appendectomies, hysterectomies) can be quite risky, if not entirely unnecessary. The results of the study point to a continued lack of understanding about IBS, what it is, how to test for it, and how to treat it.

On average, it might take four to six years for you to receive a diagnosis of IBS, usually after undergoing a variety of costly and invasive diagnostic procedures. This type of diagnosis of exclusion also costs patients in other ways, including extra costs for more prescriptions, more over-the-counter medications, and more days off work for tests and doctors' appointments. And this is not to mention the emotional and financial toll of multiple tests and co-pays. We've had patients who spent $20,000 in out-of-pocket co-pays for a variety of investigations before the diagnosis of IBS was finally settled on.

IBS and Women

Statistically, many IBS patients are women, which is why IBS has long been considered a "women's disease." Regardless of the statistics, both men and women with IBS suffer equally.

As recently as the 1980s, more than a few physicians, including gastroenterologists, dismissively spread the idea that IBS was not an actual disease, but a mental disorder, a hysteria among women who were nervous, anxious, or "hormonal." Women could become so nervous that they couldn't control their guts. Or maybe IBS was an off-shoot of their periods, menopause, or hormones. Only a few years ago, we heard a doctor outlining these beliefs as if they were medical truth to a room full of doctors about to sit for their gastrointestinal boards.

Even though we now know that none of this is true, the bias has staying power. It continues to linger and support the all-too-common belief that any chronic disease is related first and foremost to a person's mental state. This is what we were told in medical school and in residency as recently as 20 years ago. "Those IBS patients you're going to see? They're all nuts!" These were the beliefs of some of our peers and even our mentors.

This attitude shows how IBS has been misrepresented, and why so many of our patients come to us in extreme physical and emotional distress. After having been poked and prodded, they feel as if no one believes what they're feeling and what they're going through. What's worse, they doubt their ability to sense the state of their own bodies. They've had test after test and yet the results always come back negative or inconclusive, leaving them in much the same bewildered state that they were in before the tests.

From our perspective, and to put it bluntly, IBS is *not* a "women's disease."

Anxiety Doesn't Give You IBS— IBS Gives You Anxiety

"My family thinks I'm crazy."
"They think I'm doing all this for attention."
"They think I'm just stressing myself so much that I'm making myself sick."

This is another common refrain we hear from our patients. Again, none of this is true. It's not all in your head and you can't fix IBS by avoiding stress. There *is* a medical reason for your symptoms, and we're getting better at diagnosing and treating your symptoms. Australia's University of Newcastle professors Nicholas Talley and Marjorie Walker have written, "Being anxious can give you gut problems, but having gut problems can make you anxious." Or as they concluded in one of their recent studies of two-thirds of patients with anxiety, the disease drives the anxiety. The anxiety does *not* create the disease.

Thankfully, in the past 15 years, most of these beliefs about IBS have begun to fade, lessening the stigma, the misinformation, and the lack of compassion. As we continue to make progress in understanding IBS—how it originates, what keeps it going, and most importantly, how to treat it effectively—the cloud of anxiety around it will evaporate.

In the next chapter, we review the anatomy of the digestive system, describe how the normal gut breaks down and moves food, and what can go wrong in the process.

CHAPTER 2

Getting to Know Your Gut

N ow that we've covered the symptoms and history of IBS, including how it's regarded within and outside the medical community, we can move on to the gut itself—your gastrointestinal system.

In order to understand why you have IBS, you need to know how your gut both succeeds and fails to protect you. This involves the *microbiome*, which varies throughout the gut. It is critical to understand the microbiome and how it relates to IBS. In this chapter we use a step-by-step approach to help you understand the gut's functions, and we answer questions such as:

How does the normal digestive system work?

How does food move through the gut?

Where are the various types of bacteria in the gut?

How does the immune system protect the gut?

Your Gut Feelings

When you go to the doctor's office complaining of bloating, what does that mean? Do you have excessive flatulence? Are you concerned because your abdomen protrudes? Do you belch often? Depending on the answers to these—and other—questions, your diagnosis and treatment will differ.

Imagine your gut as a car engine. When you take your car to the shop because the engine is knocking, the mechanic has to figure out which of the car's multiple components could be the cause. Similarly, depending on your gastrointestinal symptoms, the doctor has to identify the parts of your gut that may be malfunctioning. And just as your car's electrical system can go haywire, the gut's circuitry, which acts as a type of switchboard or communication center to and from the brain, can become disconnected as well.

A mechanic typically uses a computer to pinpoint the car's issue. But the gut can only tell you that something is wrong in four main ways: bloating, pain, vomiting (nausea) and diarrhea, or constipation. That doesn't give the doctor a lot of information.

The doctor has to dissect and qualify these symptoms. For example, is your bloating related only to meals, or do you feel bloated day and night? Only after extensive questioning about the timing, intensity, severity, and pattern of your symptoms can the doctor unravel your digestive condition.

Your Digestive System

To make a diagnosis, the doctor considers the entire digestive system. Your gut is not just a simple tube that absorbs food, breaks it down, and turns it into waste. It's far more complex, as it's associated with many functions and diseases. We won't examine the vast array of digestive diseases in this book, but we'll explore the function of each section of the gut, and describe how each relates to the microbiome.

The gut can be broken down into various parts (Table 2.1). The hollow organs that make up the digestive system include the mouth, esophagus, stomach, small intestine, large intestine, and anus. The pancreas, liver, and gallbladder (although the gallbladder is not exactly solid) are the solid organs of the GI tract, and we will take a look at the appendix as well. Each organ can contribute to bloating, pain, vomiting and diarrhea, or constipation, depending on the disease. Yes, even a disease that primarily affects the esophagus can cause constipation. For example, Chagas disease, which is related to an infection with the parasite *Trepanosoma cruzi*, provokes the esophagus to stop working and may cause constipation as well. The primary symptoms of this infection relate to swallowing, but constipation provides a clue.

YOUR MOUTH

The first point of contact with the digestive system is your mouth, where food begins the journey of digestion. When you think about eating, your brain tells your gut, "Get ready, food is coming." This turns on the production of saliva, which contains enzymes to begin the breakdown of food. It also lubricates the food and helps you taste it. At the same time, the brain sends signals to your stomach and to the colon via the *vagus nerve*. The signals flip a switch to convert the digestive system from fasting state ("cleaning mode") to feeding state ("grinding and digesting mode"). You'll see how important this is when we discuss SIBO and food choices later in the book.

The vagus nerve signals also ramp up the pancreas to secrete digestive juices and insulin, the stomach to produce more acid, and the gallbladder to squeeze out bile to help liquify fats and add more blood flow to the gut to gather up nutrients.

The act of looking at food functions more like a dimmer switch than an on-off signal to eat. When you take your first bite of food, the vagus nerve in your brain is excited, and as you swallow it becomes even more excited. By the time the food reaches your stomach, it's really excited. The brain signals increase in intensity as the food moves closer to the small intestine, where absorption occurs.

As it relates to the gut, the microbiome begins in the mouth, as it contains about 10 billion bacteria. You may have heard that "the human mouth is the dirtiest place in the body." The word "dirty" suggests that bacteria in the mouth are infectious. That's a great line for mouthwash commercials, but in reality the microorganisms—or microbes—throughout the human body are healthy when in balance and unhealthy when the balance is disrupted. Yes, your mouth is teeming with bacteria, but most of it is harmless or even necessary for health.

The microbes found in the human mouth have developed over time through evolution. Although you may swallow some of those mouth bacteria with your food, most of them don't survive the acid bath in your stomach. This means of protection prevents the mouth bacteria from affecting the stomach, which has its own microbiome.

Table 2.1 Selected functions of the digestive system. Note that mucus production and formation of biofilm occur throughout the GI tract.

Mouth/Pharynx	• Saliva production
	• Mastication (chewing)
	• Communicating with the brain to kickstart digestion in the GI tract
	• Transferring food to the esophagus without allowing the food to enter the lungs
	• Harboring the oral microbiome
Esophagus	• Actively transferring food to the stomach
	• Keeping the stomach contents from refluxing into the mouth and lungs
	• Harboring the esophageal microbiome
Stomach	• Temporarily storing food during the feeding phase
	• Grinding the food via strong contractions
	• Producing acid
	• Producing enzymes and some hormones
	• Controlling the rate and volume of food introduced to the small bowel
	• Note that it doesn't have a significant role in absorption (except water, alcohol, and some drugs)
	• Harboring the gastric microbiome

Small intestine	• A major part of the immune system
	• Main site of digestion and absorption of food via enzymes
	• Producing hormones to regulate the GI tract
	• Moving the small intestine contents to the colon
	• Harboring the small intestine microbiome
Large intestine	• Absorbing excess water
	• Acting as a stool reservoir
	• Harboring stool and the colonic microbiome
Pancreas	• Producing pancreatic enzymes
	• Producing bicarbonate to neutralize stomach acid
	• Producing various hormones, including insulin
Liver	• A major part of the immune system
	• Performing detoxification
	• Producing bile
	• Producing, regulating, and storing many vital hormones, chemicals, and elements
	• Destroying aging blood cells
Gallbladder	• Storing gall (another name for bile)

YOUR ESOPHAGUS

The esophagus is a muscular tube that serves as a conduit for food from the mouth to the stomach. Through a coordinated series of muscular contractions—a process called peristalsis—the esophagus moves the food into the stomach where a valve, or sphincter, acts as a gateway to keep the food from going back up into the esophagus.

Functionally, the esophagus is vital to health. If your esophagus functions poorly, you may struggle to eat and maintain good nutrition. The esophagus has its own microbiome that has not, as yet, been fully characterized.

YOUR STOMACH

The next stop for nutrients is the stomach, a muscular organ that is critical to digestion. The stomach doesn't just hold food; it mixes and grinds it. Think of the stomach as one of those old-fashioned metal meat grinders. The top of the stomach holds the food in a reservoir and the bottom third grinds the food. The stomach's churning motion helps convert the now mushed-up food mixed with acid into a liquid called *chyme*, and slowly empties its contents into the small intestine.

The stomach also secretes a large volume of acidic fluid—two liters, or a half gallon, a day. The acid, which serves multiple purposes, has a very low pH and is strong enough to eat through a sheet of steel. Acid will kill bacteria (less than 100 per mL bacteria appear in the stomach) and prevent viruses from entering the small intestine. Acid also plays an important role in denaturing proteins—that is, it unfolds proteins to make them easier to break down later on in the digestive process.

The elaborate grinding of the stomach squeezes and mashes food until it can move through the *pyloric sphincter*—the valve between the stomach and the small intestine. This sphincter stays tight as the grinding motions move food from the top to the bottom of the stomach. The pylorus won't allow food pieces bigger than 1 mm (the size of a pinhead) to enter the small bowel during this phase.

Remarkably, during the grinding process, the stomach and small intestine "talk" to each other. The stomach may be full of food, but it will stop grinding if the small intestine isn't ready to receive more food. Only when the small intestine says, "Send more food," does the stomach resume emptying.

Remember, the gut has two modes: feeding (digestion) and fasting (cleaning). Two to four hours after you eat and digest a meal, the feeding mode turns off and fasting mode begins. It takes about two hours to digest carbohydrates, and about four hours to digest heavy fatty food or high-protein food. During the fasting mode, waves of electrical activity induce the gut to sweep residual undigested material through the digestive tract. This "housekeeping" role is known as the *migrating motor complex*. Most often, but not always, this procedure begins in the stomach.

The migrating motor complex is a series of quick repetitive contractions that move along the gut. The process is exactly like sweeping a floor: you make five to ten brush strokes in one place, then move a little further along, repeat and move along again. The whole event lasts for about five to eight minutes before moving down the gut. The muscular contractions push the material into the small intestine, stripping out debris and other indigestible particulates. After the event is over, the wave disappears for about 90 minutes and then reappears every 90 minutes until the next meal. When you eat again, the cycle of digestion and cleaning repeats itself.

YOUR SMALL INTESTINE

After the partially digested food passes through the pyloric sphincter into the small intestine (also known as the small bowel), wavelike contractions called *peristaltic waves* mix digestive juices with the food as it moves through the small intestine.

The small intestine consists of three parts: the *duodenum* (the first section), the *jejunum* (the middle area), and the *ileum* (the end section). Even though it's called the small intestine, it's a very long organ, measuring up to 20 feet long, and its accordion-like ridges create a greater surface area. In addition, its inner lining contains small hair-like projections—called *villi*—that further increase the surface area. If you stretched out the small intestine and its villi, it would cover the surface area of a tennis court!

The duodenum—usually about 10 inches long—receives the partially digested food from the stomach and further digests it so that it can be better absorbed in the rest of the small intestine (the jejunum and the ileum). Food from the stomach, bile from the liver, and digestive juices from the pancreas converge in the duodenum. The bile ducts from the liver connect to the duodenum to deliver bile. The pancreas also sends its juices to the duodenum. Together with other secretions from the gallbladder and small intestine, this mix of enzymes helps the body digest food and absorb nutrients.

The jejunum, which averages eight feet in length, further aids in absorbing water and other nutrients—mostly sugars, amino acids, and fatty acids. The ileum (measuring about 11 feet) at the end of the small intestine absorbs the bile acid and Vitamin B 12. It connects to the *cecum,* the first part of the *colon* (large intestine), via the *ileocecal valve.*

The ileocecal valve has an important role in separating the colon microbiome from that of the small intestine, which contains less than 1000 bacteria per mL. As with any other valve in the human body, it may not function properly, occasionally causing the contents of the colon to reflux back into the small intestine. The small intestine, however, resists by using its peristaltic waves. Similarly, stomach acid can reflux into the esophagus, waking up the esophagus to push the acid back into the stomach. Gastrointestinal problems can occur when the movement of the small intestine or the esophagus is unable to push the reflux material back where it belongs.

YOUR COLON

The large intestine, which drapes like a scarf around the small intestine, includes the *appendix,* the *colon,* and the *rectum.* If you were to look down at your midsection from above, you would see a four- to five-foot-long muscular tube that begins on the lower right side of your body, in the lower right quadrant of your abdomen. The ascending colon rises and crosses over to the left part of your lower midsection via the transverse colon, drops down again via the descending colon, curves upward just a little via the sigmoid colon, drops straight down again into the rectum, and finally, into the anus. The ascending colon heads toward the liver; the descending colon flows into the rectum and anus.

The colon is a social organ; more than 1000 different types of bacteria live there. Of the many trillions of bacteria in the human microbiome, the largest proportion of these bacteria is located in the colon, which harbors about 1 trillion bacteria, as well as fungi (fungus) and viruses. The many bacteria that inhabit the colon can further aid digestion. This is the beginning of a conversation about gut bacteria.

Overall, the major function of the colon is to absorb the last bit of excess water from the material leaving the small intestine, process waste products from the body, and, through peristalsis, help move the stool into the rectum to be eliminated. In effect, the colon acts as the gut's "dryer," absorbing remaining water and electrolytes. About 10 liters of liquid pass through the small intestine every day, whereas only about half a liter passes through the colon. More than 90 percent of the water is absorbed in the small intestine.

Interestingly, you can live without a colon, but you can't live without a small intestine. So why do humans have a colon? Through evolution, mammals developed colons to be able to defecate on demand. When we needed to hold our stool in, we could. For example, early man could be quiet for safety and security or keep moving in search of food or to flee a predator. The ability to hold in stool gave mammals a huge advantage over other animals.

YOUR RECTUM AND ANUS

The *rectum* resides at the lower end of the GI tract. This straight-down extension of the sigmoid colon connects to the anus. The rectum stores feces until it pushes the stool into the anus and out of your body during a bowel movement. The rectum senses stool and tells you when things are ready to pass out. The function of the rectum and anus is extraordinary, in that it can hold a mixture of water, solids, and gas yet it can let the gas out separately. In some patients with IBS, the rectum over-senses stool. If it detects a lower volume of stool too early, you may have the feeling of urgency. This is referred to as rectal hypersensitivity.

YOUR PANCREAS

The oblong-shaped *pancreas* is located behind the stomach in the upper left abdomen. It converts food and other nutrients into fuel for the body, and produces pancreatic juice that enters the duodenum of the small intestine. The digestive enzymes secreted by the pancreas help break down proteins, carbohydrates, and fats. The pancreas also produces the hormones *insulin* and *glucagon* to help regulate blood sugar. Finally, the pancreas secretes bicarbonate that neutralizes the stomach acid. A balanced pH in the small bowel is crucial for the function of mucosal cells and digestive enzymes.

YOUR LIVER

The *liver*, the largest solid organ in the body, is found in the upper right quadrant of your midsection, just above the colon. It plays an important role in the body's immune system, as it is the epicenter of detoxification: it will detoxify any toxin it encounters. Alcohol is the most well-known toxin broken down—or metabolized—by the liver.

The liver also produces *bile acids*—the yellowish-brown enzymes that eliminate cholesterol from the body and aid in gut motility for digestion and absorption of fats in the small intestine. Bile acids also contribute to the color of your bowel movements.

YOUR GALLBLADDER

The *gallbladder* is a pear-shaped, hollow organ that sits just beneath the liver. In between meals, during the fasting phase, the gallbladder processes, stores, and concentrates bile from the liver. When the gut needs bile, the gallbladder squeezes the right amount out to help digest fats and other components. Once in the gut, some of the bile gets reabsorbed into the blood from the ileum, the last section of the small intestine, and recycles back into the liver.

If your gallbladder is removed or is not functioning properly, bile will flow straight from the liver into the small intestine and eventually to the colon, often resulting in diarrhea. It's important to note that when bacteria encounter bile, they convert it to toxic bile acids (such as deoxycholic acid and lithocholic acid), which are believed to cause diarrhea. This is known as *bile acid diarrhea (BAD)* and is different from SIBO, but it's worse when SIBO is present. One of the main causes of bile acid diarrhea is SIBO.

YOUR APPENDIX

The *appendix* is a tiny, worm-shaped organ that attaches to the first section of the colon in the lower right quadrant of your midsection. The appendix was long thought to be an unnecessary vestige of our evolutionary past, but lately it's been hypothesized that the appendix acts as a storehouse for the gut's healthy bacterial composition, and it may play a crucial role in the immune system. For example, we have shown that the appendix has an important role in the balance of methane-producing gut microbes.

GUT OR GI MOTILITY

Digestion requires constant, synchronized contractions of the various gut muscles to control the movement of food through the gastrointestinal tract. These contractions are known as *gut motility*. Motility problems can develop when the nerves and/or muscles of the gut are not working properly. Abnormal gut motility can lead to bloating, pain, nausea, and diarrhea or constipation, all of the symptoms related to IBS. If you suffer from IBS with constipation, your intestinal movements may be too slow, while if you suffer from IBS with diarrhea, your gut may propel its contents too fast. This is not a universal rule, however. If your bowels are extremely slow, you may have diarrhea, and if they are fast, but not coordinated properly, this may lead to constipation.

The Feeding Phase

When gut motility is working well, during the feeding phase the stomach pushes food mixed with acid toward the pylorus, which senses whether the food is broken down enough to allow it to pass into the small intestine. The small intestine is responsible for mixing and spreading the food to maximize protein and sugar break down, as well as mixing fats and bile into little packages during the feeding phase. When the stomach is full of food and distends, the *gastrocolic reflex* signals the colon to empty, and the colon pushes stool forward. This is why you occasionally have a bowel movement after eating. The reflex also functions to drive the existing intestinal contents through the gastrointestinal tract to help make way for ingested food.

The very act of eating can provoke an overreaction of this reflex in some patients with IBS because of their heightened visceral (intestinal) sensitivity. IBS patients tend to describe the experience of pain within the internal organs (the viscera) at a more intense level than normal, leading to the classic symptoms of IBS.

The Fasting Phase

After the feeding phase ends, the fasting phase begins. Initially the small bowel doesn't move or only partially moves such that food gets mixed with enzymes in the small intestine. When digestion is complete, housekeeper cleaning waves (also known as migrating motor complexes phase 3) begin and occur every 90 to 120 minutes for a few minutes at a time (Figure 2.1). The waves move into the small intestine, where they push the remnants of undigested food, bowel secretions, and excess bacteria forward and dump them into the colon.

The housekeeper function is one of the keys to understanding IBS. For those who are significantly affected by IBS, the housekeeping role malfunctions and "cleaning" of the bowel is impaired; that is, more bacteria accumulate and grow on the debris in the small intestine, producing many side-products—including gas—which leads to bloating, abdominal distension, diarrhea, or constipation.

In a clinical study published in 2002, we found that IBS and SIBO patients had 60 percent fewer housekeeping waves compared to healthy controls, meaning that the small bowel motility of these IBS patients was insufficient to completely clean out their small intestine. On a regular basis, bacteria in the colon creep back up to the small intestine in search of more food. However, the small intestine pushes them back to the colon with housekeeper waves. If these waves are impaired, bacteria can build up in the small intestine. This is also known as *small intestinal bacterial overgrowth (SIBO)*. SIBO can lead to fermentation and the production of gases, including hydrogen sulfide, methane, and hydrogen, as well as other by-products, leading to multiple symptoms that include brain fog, diarrhea or constipation, and fatigue.

One of the main pillars of IBS treatment includes medications to strengthen and promote the housekeeper waves. Chemicals called neurotransmitters interact with receptors in the small intestine to facilitate contractions that propagate the housekeeper waves and move food in an organized fashion. Drugs that boost these neurotransmitters, such as serotonin agonists and erythromycin, can activate smooth muscles in the small intestine to move the food through the gastrointestinal tract. These drugs will be discussed in more detail later.

Gut motility also plays an important role during movement of the stool in the colon and eventual defecation. The anal sphincter has an external voluntary muscle with an internal involuntary muscle on top of it. Stool moves down to the rectum, which distends. This sends a signal to the internal sphincter to relax and get ready to push the stool out through muscular contractions. When the internal sphincter relaxes, the rectum distends a little and the waste material moves to the end of the rectum and close to the anus. At this point, your body senses if it's filled with gas or if it's liquid or solid. If it's gas, then you let it go through flatulence by relaxing the external sphincter (in socially acceptable situations). If it's liquid, you know you need to hurry to the bathroom. If it's solid, you know that if you want, you can hold it until later.

Those of you with IBS with diarrhea and SIBO may have altered ability to accurately sense the amount and consistency of waste in the rectum. Up to 30 percent of SIBO/IBS patients have smearing or fecal incontinence; that is, they are unable to control their bowel movements, causing stool (fecal matter) to leak unexpectedly from the rectum. This happens in both men and women, but it's more common in women. Even more notable, patients with IBS and SIBO have altered stool form. The stool is more

Figure 2.1 High resolution image of migrating motor complex (housekeeper waves).

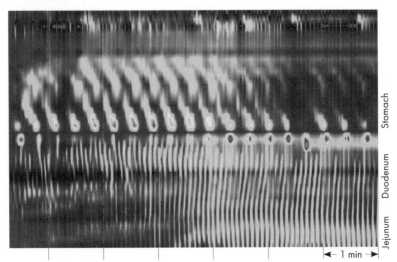

like peanut butter, and it you've had peanut butter on your hands, you know how hard it is to remove. So, if stool like that passes through the anus, it's hard to clean and sometimes it cannot be completely cleaned by just wiping after bowel movements.

Gut Immunity

Motility issues can also stem from problems in gut immunity. Your gut has millions of immune cells—more immune cells than anywhere else in your body. The intestinal immune system encounters more antigens—toxins or other foreign substances that induce an immune response—than any other part of the body. That's because you're bringing the outside world into your body by eating. You need defenses.

Your gut is also the home of the body's largest *microbiome*. This microbiome ideally contains a healthy balance of bacteria, as well as fungi, parasites, viruses, and archaea (single-cell organisms, including methanogens, which produce methane gas as a metabolic by-product). These microbes live throughout your digestive system. They live in your mouth and in your intestines, and they have different functions and interactions. If the delicate balance of the microbiome is upset, for example, by food poisoning or excessive bacteria in the small intestine, you may develop IBS.

One of the most complicated components of the gut's immune system is *GALT*—the *gut-associated lymphoid tissue*, a key defense system that's part of the mucosa-associated lymphoid tissue. Lymphoid tissue is part of the body's immune system that is important for immune response and helps protect it from infection and foreign bodies. Lymphoid tissues cover most of the intestines and monitor almost everything that passes through. In addition, they detect and attack gut invaders. Finally, the lymphoid tissues produce antibodies, one of the body's main lines of defense against bacteria and viruses.

The largest collection of lymphoid tissue resides in the small intestine, where the gut reacts to what you eat. The small intestine has a permeable surface that allows food to enter your digestive system, and it's also where many forms of food-poisoning bacteria multiply. For example, we now know that food poisoning can trigger IBS. We'll discuss this recently discovered cause of IBS in Chapter 4.

Immunity Defenders

Many disease-causing organisms enter the body through the mucous membranes that cover the intestines, so it's vital for the gut-associated lymphoid tissues to provide an effective immune response when necessary. Although the epithelial cells that line the intestinal tract comprise a single cell layer, they form a barrier against the penetration of microbes. Epithelial cells of the small intestine can interact with and trap bacteria in the mucus. They also sense microorganisms and secrete chemicals to respond to the entry of bacteria. In addition, mucosal cells of the intestine only allow microorganisms to enter through them and not in-between them. This is due to the chain links—known as tight junctions—that connect the mucosal cells. Many diseases can affect tight junctions (also known as "leaky gut") that allow the unscreened bacteria to enter the body.

Another key component of the mucosal immune response to gut antigens and bacteria are *Peyer's patches*. These immune sensors are small masses of lymphoid nodules found throughout the ileum, at the end of the small intestine. They play an important role in the gut's immune system by monitoring populations of intestinal bacteria and preventing the growth of disease-causing bacteria in the intestines.

Differences in Immunity

Your adult immune system is entirely different from what it was when you were a child. A child is born with an immature, innate immune system. As the child grows, the immune system matures, adapts, and acquires memory. In addition to fighting bacteria, viruses, fungi, and parasites, the immune system assumes other roles, as well, such as tissue repair, wound healing, elimination of dead cells and cancer cells, and formation of a healthy gut microbiome.

Everything you eat affects your microbiome. Various dietary patterns shape the microbiome and can lead to differences in immunity. For example, the gut immune systems of children in a developing country—who may contract gut diseases at an early age—develop differently than the gut immune systems of American children. This is because the types of microbes found in the microbiome in the developing world are different from those in the United States.

Table 2.2 Natural protective factors against SIBO.

Phase III migrating motor complexes (housekeeper waves)
Antimicrobial effects of bile acid and pancreatic secretions
Ileocecal valve
Stomach acid

Gut problems may occur when there are bacteria your immune system has never seen before. If you eat a meal in a developing country, you might experience gastrointestinal upset. Similarly, someone from an underdeveloped country who comes to the United States may become sick from eating a fast-food hamburger. Disrupting the delicate balance of your microbiome can lead to gastrointestinal symptoms and potential significant discomfort.

As you've learned, the gut is complicated but highly effective. Table 2.2 lists the natural defenses the gut has to protect itself from SIBO. In the next chapter, we'll discuss the basics of the microbiome and its associated diseases.

CHAPTER 3

The Gut Microbiome: Your Second Self

"We cannot fathom the marvelous complexity of an organic being. . . . Each living creature must be looked at as a microcosm—a little universe, formed of a host of self-propagating organisms, inconceivably minute and as numerous as the stars in heaven."
—Charles Darwin, 1850

The gut microbiome is currently one of the hottest topics in the healthcare and medical industry, as researchers continue to uncover surprising connections between the gut microbiome and many aspects of health. The gut microbiome can potentially be considered a completely separate organ in the body, as it contains a vast ecosystem of bacteria, viruses, fungi, and protozoa. This delicate ecosystem can be thrown out of balance, however, and may worsen or lead to chronic diseases such as heart disease, diabetes, and cancer. Furthermore, many other chronic diseases, including obesity, Parkinson's disease, inflammatory bowel disease (IBD), mood disorders, liver disease, and, of course, irritable bowel syndrome (IBS) may actually be microbiome diseases.

A more diverse gut microbiome can lead to a more robust, adaptable immune system. The wide variety of protective bacterial strains already found in your gut were partly passed down from your mother at childbirth.

Antibiotics, diet, infections, and other factors may reduce their abundance, but these bacteria are usually not completely eradicated. It's important to nurture and reinforce a healthy gut microbiome.

There are numerous beneficial functions of a healthy gut microbiome. Gut microbes modulate other bacteria and facilitate the extraction and fermentation of dietary fibers. They generate heat and can change your basal metabolic rate. They also produce vitamins and are mediators of peptides (small proteins), which play key roles in regulating the activities of other molecules, modulating immune responses, and influencing other bacteria.

The way in which the microbiome interacts with the body is important to gastrointestinal function. The human microbiome produces some of the same compounds that are produced by human cells. For example, the microbiome secretes *serotonin*, a mood chemical, leading some researchers to believe that bacteria can influence mood as well as insulin-like proteins and other chemicals that allow your body to function. Serotonin has a neuromodulating effect that causes nerves to fire and modulate gut function. A disruption in the microbiome may increase serotonin levels and can lead to diarrhea, or, if hormone production is reduced, constipation.

The microbiome can be modified and used to your benefit or to your harm. For example, if you receive the microbiome of an obese person through a fecal transplant, you may become obese. If you receive methanogen-producing microbes through a fecal transplant, you may become severely constipated. On the positive side, if you have a resistant infection with *Clostridoides difficile (C. difficile)*, a fecal transplant is as likely to resolve it as would antibiotic treatment.

Your Bacterial Tribe

Your gut is home to trillions of bacteria, viruses, and fungi that congregate collectively to comprise your microbiome. This large gastrointestinal tribe shapes the onset, incidence, and treatment of a startling number of diseases. In the past 20 years since microbiome research began, much has been discovered about how this unseen ecosystem interacts with all aspects of human life, and the rate of discovery shows no signs of slowing. Our greater understanding of the microbiome is helping explore the intricacies of diet, metabolic disorders, cancer treatment, and more.

A Brief History of the Microbiome

The existence of the normal microbiome is ancient and ever-present. In fact, humans are vehicles for the preservation and growth of these microbes, and we are actually more bacterial than human. Try to imagine that you are bacteria in soil: you have to move around to find food, fight with other bacteria, and look for the ideal temperatures to grow (too cold and you can't multiply; too hot and you'll die). Furthermore, the sun's UV light can kill you. In the human body, you have all the food you need, there's no light, and it's always the perfect temperature (37°C/98.6°F).

Until recently, scientists believed that less than half of the body was made of human cells and the rest bacteria. Now we believe there are at least as many bacteria as human cells in the body, and there may even be up to 10 times more bacteria. You may be host to almost 100 trillion microbes! One kilogram, or more than two pounds, of your body weight is made up of these microbes. One gram of stool has 100 billion microbes in it, and half of them are dead. There are over 1000 known species of bacteria in the human gut microbiome, and each has the potential to play a different role in your body.

The microbiome also exists in different parts of the body: on your skin and in your mouth, gut, and vagina. The largest microbiome by far is in your gut. In Chapter 2, we explained that each organ in the gut harbors different amounts of bacteria and, as we'll explore later in this chapter, different types of bacteria. Most of the bacteria are extremely important for your health, while others may cause disease.

What Is a Microbiome?

Your microbiome is a collection of microbes—bacteria, archaea (ancient single-celled organisms), fungi, and viruses. Sometimes they help each other, and other times they compete with each other. There are even viruses that can kill or modify bacteria. We call the collection of these microbes, including their more than 3 million genes (150 times more than human genes), the *microbiota*. Today the technical terms microbiota and microbiome are used interchangeably.

The word microbiome combines the word "micro," meaning small, and "biome," meaning a major ecological community. The term microbiome was coined in 2003, so the study of the microbiome is a relatively new science. The Human Microbiome Project, sponsored by the National Institutes of Health, was an effort to define the contents of a microbiome. In 2007, the Human Microbiome Project published a paper in the journal *Nature* illustrating that the microbiome encompasses all zones of the body.

Scientists first began to examine the gut microbiome in the stool, it being easy to obtain a stool sample. They used the stool as a surrogate for the entire 25 feet of the gut, not realizing that stool is only the gut's exit material. We now know that the microbiome in the 20-foot-long small intestine is radically different from the microbiome in the stool. Declaring that the stool represents the microbiome in the gut is incomplete and incorrect. In a recent paper (2020), we published for the first time the bacterial profile of the entire small intestine and colon (represented by stool). Even at the highest levels, the small bowel's profile is completely different. We now know that there's no way to know what's happening in the longest part of the gut simply by testing stool.

What's more, the microbiome in the small intestine may be considered eminently more important than the microbiome in the stool. The interaction between the microbiome and the large absorbing surface area of the small intestine may indicate how some people become diabetic or obese. More importantly, for the purposes of this book, small intestine bacterial overgrowth (SIBO) and IBS-related symptoms are directly related to how your microbiome reacts in the small intestine. That's why we primarily focus on the small intestine when examining the microbiome.

We've developed a technique that inserts an instrument called an endoscope into the mouth and snakes it down into the small intestine. Then, using a newly designed sterile aspiration catheter, we remove samples from different parts of the small intestine. Although it's much more difficult to collect samples from the small intestine, we've found it's worth it in order to examine its microbiome. When studying the small intestinal microbiome, it's critical to collect the sample, process it, and culture it correctly.

Unfortunately, this doesn't usually happen in most medical centers. You can't just suction juice from the small intestine and send it to a central lab that processes and reports it like a urine culture (greater than or less than 100,000 bacteria). A recent study by Dr. Brian Lacy from Mayo Clinic showed that 20 percent of samples using this approach are useless because they are contaminated with mouth bacteria. In the last three to four years, we've studied and validated the techniques for obtaining the small bowel microbiome fluid, processing and culturing the thick fluid, and culturing and deep sequencing the whole microbiome, thus creating a gold standard.

Envision the Microbiome as a Large Active City

Imagine a vast microbiome city in your small intestine. This city has many inhabitants with different jobs—plumbers, doctors, and sanitation workers among them. As long as the city's microbiome system stays in balance and remains diverse, the city functions well. But if you take an antibiotic and fire all the sanitation workers, the city fills with trash. In a similar analogy, taking probiotics is like adding 1 million doctors every day, and that can throw the city out of whack as well. Any disturbance in the city has an effect on the rest of the microbiome.

Collectively, the microbiome acts in your defense. If you're a big city, it's difficult for an invading army to penetrate the city walls. A well-balanced microbiome makes it hard for infections to grab hold. Think of a balanced microbiome as a set of niches, with each niche represent-ing a home. In the homes are different types of bacteria. If one home is empty, there's room for an interloper. For example, the microbiome pro-tects against infections from *C. difficile*, which has become a scourge in hospitals because it's largely resistant to antibiotics. If you take antibiotics to reduce infection, they also reduce the number of defenders in your city. In this weakened environment, *C. difficile* finds a niche (or home), grows there and can become harmful to the colon, which may lead to colitis. Other invading opportunistic organisms can take advantage of the damaged city and overrun it, much like a coup.

Microbiome Components Specific to Health

Your microbiome contains five specific components that promote health and ward off disease.

Diversity of bacteria and fungi in the gut. In the large microbiome city of your gut, the more diverse the population, the healthier it is. You wouldn't want a city filled only with doctors or lawyers, for example.

Distribution of bacteria and fungi. Differing types of bacteria are positioned strategically throughout the gut. For example, the colon bacteria are different from the small intestine bacteria because accumulation of bacteria from the colon in the small intestine leads to SIBO and its associated symptoms.

Number and composition of bacteria. In the scientific literature this is described as relative or absolute abundance. With thousands of varieties of bacteria, your microbiome city has occupants with characteristics that allow them to complete their specific tasks. The number of each microbe is proportional to its roles and functions. Five plumbers would not be enough for a big city. You need the right amount of each bacterium for functioning harmony.

Products of bacteria. The many inhabitants of your microbiome city produce a wide variety of products, some of which are good and others are bad. For example, some bacteria have properties that reduce inflammation in the gut and others promote normal motility. On the other hand, gas and other chemicals produced by bacteria in the microbiome can contribute to the symptoms of IBS. It's important to understand that bacteria are not "good" or "bad" all the time. It's more about maintaining balance in your microbiome.

Resiliency. If you look at your microbiome after taking antibiotics, you'll likely find that the numbers of microorganisms are drastically reduced. Two weeks later, the bacteria repopulate your gut and the microbiome snaps back to normal. That's resiliency. But if you continue to take courses of antibiotics, they can adversely affect your microbiome. The microbiome is like an elastic band that becomes a little less stretchy every time you pull on it. It may not snap back all the way if you take too many antibiotics.

What Is a "Normal" Microbiome?

Researchers have shifted their thinking from isolating and identifying the microbes in the gut to understanding their function as it relates to human health. Given that there are more than 1000 species in the human microbiome, there's a significant amount of redundancy in species function, which can be a good thing. Diseases like obesity, IBD, IBS, and diabetes have been associated with a decrease in microbial diversity. It's important to understand that there's no single normal profile of gut microbiome. Metropolitan cities share a lot of similarities, but they're not exactly the same. Let's explore this in more detail.

So, when do bacteria first manifest in the human body? We now understand that even a fetus possesses a rudimentary microbiome. Bacteria are thought to transfer through the placenta to the fetus, and have been found in the amniotic fluid of mice. Bacteria in humans have been isolated and detected in the umbilical cord blood without any evidence of infection or inflammation. The human placenta harbors its own microbiome, and surprisingly, a healthy baby's first stool is not sterile. Vaginal birth or delivery by C-section can have a significant impact on the early days of colonization in the guts of newborns. Vaginal delivery is believed to more quickly prime the colonization of the gut with healthy bacteria.

By the age of three years, your gut microbiome begins to resemble your adult microbiome. Because we are skipping many colonization steps here, it's important to understand that your microbiome remains dynamic throughout your life. For example, our research shows that methanogenic archaea increase by almost five-fold from childhood into the eighth decade of life. So, even in old age, the microbiome continues to change with you. Whether this is good or bad remains to be understood.

Actually, we don't know what a "normal" microbiome looks like. Your microbiome is unique to you. There are common classic patterns, but each of us has a distinct microbiome. Your diet, environment, medications, and genetics influence your microbiome, and even your pets can affect your microbiome!

Our salient point is that there's no such thing as a "normal" microbiome; in fact, we don't know what a perfect microbiome should be. There's no known magic mix of bacteria, which makes treatment of the microbiome complicated.

In addition, your diet makes your microbiome unique. If you live in Africa, your microbiome would be different because the African diet is different from the American diet. In Greece, people eat Greek food exclusively, and in Africa, they eat regional foods. However, in North America, we may eat Greek food one night, Italian food another night, and Mexican food the next night. As Americans, many of us tend to eat different types of cuisine every night. Never in our history has our diet been so diverse, and this factor is likely modifying our microbiome as well.

Food additives can also disrupt the microbiome. For example, emulsifiers are added to food to make it creamy, or sodium benzoate is added to reduce fungal growth and preserve shelf life. These additives make food more appealing, but they have the potential to disrupt the microbiome. An emulsifier such as polysorbate 80 disrupts mucous membranes and, in effect, emulsifies your microbiome too. And sodium benzoate kills fungi that are supposed to be in the microbiome.

Different Organs, Different Microbiomes

As we mentioned in Chapter 2, each of the gut components has its own microbiome. The most common bacteria in the stool are *bacteroidetes* and *firmicutes;* however the bacterial composition in the stool microbiome varies widely—from 10 percent to 90 percent—which is why we can't rely on stool testing to characterize the gut microbiome.

The small intestine has its own unique microbiome composition. In the new REIMAGINE study, we examined aspirates from the small intestine to define for the first time the composition of the small intestine's microbiome. We now know that this microbiome consists of two major groups of bacteria: *firmicutes* and *proteobacteria.*

We also discovered that the composition of the microbiome along the length of a person's small intestine remains relatively consistent, and is radically distinct when compared to the stool microbiome. Characterization of the small intestine's microbiome is imperative if we are to truly understand the relationship between the human microbiome and disease.

Before REIMAGINE, studies of the microbiome were not fully standardized. If a researcher sent a stool sample to two different laboratories, it might yield two different results. Fresh stool versus flash-frozen stool might produce different results as well. There was no standardized way to assess the stool microbiome. Over 18 months, we were able to streamline the process of small intestine sample collection and eventual DNA extraction to examine the microbiome.

Traditionally, there have been a variety of methods for assessing the gut microbes. The old-school method cultured a sample to watch what grew. However, the majority of microbes in the gut can't be grown in the laboratory, and therefore can't be cultured. These days bacteria and archaea are genetically sequenced. A rigorously preserved section of DNA extracted from the stool sample acts as a barcode that can be read to identify the type of microbe in the sample. Most of the time, we can amplify the DNA pieces and discern the relative frequency of bacteria in the stool. This process is called *deep sequencing*.

Sequencing, however, is not easy to perform, and the results are not always specific. Genetic sequencing can reveal the genera (groups) of bacteria and sometimes the species, but not the particular strains. One strain of *E. coli* bacterium can be quite different from another one; for example, one strain can kill and another may be harmless. Bacteria are complex and diverse.

Microbiome Diseases

When accessing the small intestine, we can combine cell culturing and genetic sequencing to test the microbiome. This process has helped strengthen the association of disruptions in the microbiome by a slew of diseases, including obesity, Parkinson's disease, *C. difficile* infections, IBD, depression and anxiety, hepatic encephalopathy, and IBS.

OBESITY

Microbiome experts are now focusing on obesity, one of the world's largest epidemics. A look at the stool microbiome reveals patterns in the ratio of bacteroidetes to firmicutes bacteria. An alteration in this ratio appears to be a signal for obesity. We also have preliminary evidence linking a specific microbe in the small intestine microbiome to obesity, and we're engaging in more research to verify this hypothesis.

We are also members of a research team examining a link between methane-producing archaea and obesity, and there appear to be two mechanisms in play. The first hypothesis is that methane produced by this microbe slows down gut transit. The slower the chyme transits, the more time the gut has to absorb nutrients. And the longer food stays in the gut, the more calories are absorbed each time you eat.

The second hypothesis focuses on the interaction of methane-producing and hydrogen-producing microbes. The methane-producing microbes need partners of another species—usually proteobacteria—to produce hydrogen. The methanogenic archaea use the hydrogen to make the methane that produces energy for them, and the loss of hydrogen can increase calories. Human cells neither produce nor use methane or hydrogen (that we know of), which are only produced by bacteria (and archaea, in the case of methane) as part of their fermentation process.

PARKINSON'S DISEASE

The microbes that populate the guts of Parkinsonian patients appear to differ from those of healthy people. This microbial difference correlates with the stooped posture and difficulty walking experienced by people with this disease.

Only a small fraction of Parkinson's disease cases is inherited. In the remainder of patients, an entity appears to kill selected nerve cells (neurons) in the brain. The prime suspect is abnormally misfolded and clumped proteins, but other possible causes include head trauma or exposure to heavy metals, pesticides, or air pollution.

One theory holds that Parkinson's disease is caused by an inflammatory reaction that alters the gut microbiome. The inflammation causes proteins, called *alpha-synuclein*, to misfold and travel along the *vagus nerve* from the lining of the gut to the brain, causing nerve cell death. A hallmark of Parkinson's disease is the presence in the brain of Lewy bodies that contain clumps of alpha-synuclein. Researchers have found signs that Lewy bodies begin to form in the colon before they manifest in the brain. This provides another hint that something in the colon may trigger or initiate the development of Parkinson's disease.

And it happens that patients with Parkinson's disease have often had digestive issues, such as constipation, long before the neurological disease appears. This can occur 2 to 10 years prior to the appearance of Parkinsonian symptoms. In our gastrointestinal motility clinic, we see many patients with constipation who have evolving Parkinson's disease.

In fact, we often diagnose Parkinson's disease for the first time in our clinic. This adds credence to the theory that Parkinson's may be a microbiome disease, inasmuch as the gastrointestinal symptoms precede the neurological symptoms.

Perhaps Parkinson's isn't a brain disease that affects the gut, but rather for some patients, a gut disease that affects the brain. Someday doctors may be able to test for microbiome changes that put people at higher risk for Parkinson's, and then restore a healthy microbe through diet or other means in order to delay or prevent the disease. Research is already underway.

CLOSTRIDIOIDES DIFFICILE

C. difficile infection is now the leading cause of hospital-based infections in the United States. This spore-forming microbe is difficult to eradicate, and it frequently recurs after treatment. The infection is strongly associated with prior use of antibiotics. Other risk factors include advanced age, immunosuppression, IBD, and use of proton pump inhibitors. These factors are all associated with changes in the composition of the gut microbiome.

Researchers have found that disturbances in the gut microbiome play a central role in *C. difficile* infections; studies show that the presence of *C. difficile* in the gut reduces microbiome diversity. *C. difficile* infections have also been associated with changes in specific microbial populations that may either protect against *C. difficile* colonization in the gut or increase susceptibility for *C. difficile* infection. In other words, if your microbiome is disturbed, you're more likely to develop a *C. difficile* infection.

Fecal Transplantation. Use of the fecal transplantation technique has been found to be a highly effective treatment for *C. difficile* infections. For recurrent infections, antibiotics are 30 percent effective, while fecal transplantation is about 90 percent effective. After a fecal transplant, the microbiome resets within two to three days. The effectiveness of microbiome fecal transplants for relapsing *C. difficile* infection is a good example of the promise this field holds. IBD, obesity, and cancer are other diseases for which fecal transplantation might be helpful, but the data are inconclusive. We'll discuss the role of fecal transplantation for IBS and SIBO in a later chapter.

INFLAMMATORY BOWEL DISEASE (IBD)

IBD includes Crohn's disease and ulcerative colitis, both chronic relapsing conditions of the gastrointestinal tract. In a patient with IBD, the bowel ulcerates, causing bleeding, strictures, and abdominal pain.

Evidence has emerged to support the gut microbiome's involvement in the development or propagation of IBD. Indeed, IBD has been associated with dramatic changes in the gut microbiome. One of the first experiments that suggested the importance of gut bacteria in IBD showed significant healing when the fecal stream was diverted. In some patients with severe refractory disease, the stool was diverted to an ostomy bag (a pouch worn to collect stool) so that no stool entered the colon. Patients' inflammation disappeared and their IBD went into remission, only to relapse when the bowel was reconnected and stool and bacteria were introduced into the colon. This phenomenon demonstrates that the mucous membranes lining the gastrointestinal tract don't become ulcerated unless they're exposed to the flow of stool and its bacteria. When stool flow was diverted back through the gut, the ulcerations and IBD symptoms returned.

Similar studies show that germ-free mice don't develop gut inflammation until bacteria are introduced. This gut inflammation is triggered or facilitated by the gut microbiome.

No single microbe has been identified as a disease-causing agent in IBD. Antibiotic treatment in Crohn's disease and ulcerative colitis shows conflicting long-term outcomes, and the use of probiotics for the treatment of IBD remains inconclusive. However, some encouraging treatment results have emerged with use of optimized microbial concoctions that include beneficial strains of bacteria.

Fecal transplantation is one of the more promising microbiome-modulating IBD therapies. Fecal transplantation studies in ulcerative colitis show improvement in remission rates; however, these studies include only small numbers of patients and use a variety of treatment methods, so they provide no definitive answers.

Clearly, gut dysbiosis plays a role in IBD. Novel therapies to treat and prevent IBD will undoubtably have to include modulation of the gut microbiome, requiring a multidimensional approach to match microbiome modulation with other therapies that target IBD and its components. Such therapies may include probiotics, prebiotics, antibiotics, and fecal transplant in a personalized approach to identify those who will benefit most.

DEPRESSION AND ANXIETY

The relationship between the gut microbiome and mental health is one of the most intriguing topics in microbiome research. Mounting evidence suggests that the gut microbiome can influence brain function via what's known as the *microbiome gut-brain axis*.

The concept of the gut-brain axis relates to the *vagus nerve*—the body's longest nerve—which runs from the brainstem to the lowest segment of the intestines. The vagus nerve is like a two-way highway, sending signals from the brain to the gut to regulate digestion as well as sending signals from the gut back to the brain. This presents a possible pathway for neurotransmitters—chemicals such as serotonin and dopamine—from the gut to receptors in the brain, where they may affect mood and behavior.

Multiple studies show how the gut microbiome influences depression. A recent Belgian study has identified two strains of bacteria that are lacking in the guts of people who've been diagnosed with depression. Other research reveals that depressed patients show decreased diversity in their gut microbiome.

Most of the current studies are based on animal models; only a few of them are human studies. More research is necessary to confirm the link between the gut microbiome and depression. Do alterations in specific species in the gut microbiome contribute to depression, or does depression induce modification of the specific species in the microbiome and eventually contribute to more severe depression? Current research on the gut microbiome and mood disorders is still in its early stages. The near future may provide answers to these questions.

HEPATIC ENCEPHALOPATHY

Hepatic encephalopathy is a condition associated with liver disease, specifically cirrhosis. It comprises a spectrum of symptoms, including difficulty thinking, personality changes, poor concentration, problems associated with handwriting or loss of other small hand movements, confusion, forgetfulness, and poor sleep. More severe symptoms are marked confusion, severe anxiety or fearfulness, disorientation regarding time and place, as well as extreme drowsiness, slowed or sluggish movement, and shaky hands or arms.

For decades, hepatic encephalopathy was believed to be related to high levels of ammonia produced by gut bacteria in the liver as a result of liver failure. Current evidence links hepatic encephalopathy to alterations in the gut microbiome. Side products of the microbiome, such as the metabolites of amino acids and toxins, superimposed on a leaky intestinal barrier may lead to hepatic encephalopathy.

Multiple mechanisms may explain defective gut functions and an altered microbiome in patients with cirrhosis. These include a delay in small intestinal motility, increased permeability of the intestinal wall, and impaired defense against bacteria and SIBO. Additionally, a decrease in bile acids may alter the gut microbiome.

Modulation of the gut microbiome may play a role in the management of hepatic encephalopathy, further establishing its connection as a microbiome disease. Lactulose, used as standard therapy in hepatic encephalopathy, works by altering the gut microbiome to decrease ammonia production and absorption. It acts as a prebiotic to increase the growth of potentially beneficial bacteria, such as *Lactobacilli*. Lactulose also acts as a laxative, which reduces overall bacterial numbers and toxins that enter the liver's blood flow. Rifaximin, a synthetic, poorly absorbed antibiotic often used to treat IBS with diarrhea, lowers the risk of bacterial resistance and is an effective treatment for hepatic encephalopathy by decreasing the bacterial load in the small intestine.

IRRITABLE BOWEL SYNDROME (IBS)

IBS is now the poster child of microbiome diseases. The rest of the microbiome-associated diseases are still in the research stage, whereas IBS is a true prototypical microbiome disease. We now have diagnostic tests (breath tests and blood tests for anti-vinculin/anti-CdtB levels) based on the gut microbiome, along with treatments that modulate the microbiome, including dietary changes and rifaximin. IBS remains the only gastrointestinal disease of the intestines for which the FDA has approved a microbiome-modulating drug (rifaximin).

Microbiome research has led to dramatic changes in the diagnosis and treatment of IBS. In the next chapter, we discuss a new cause of IBS: food poisoning.

CHAPTER 4

Food Poisoning: A New Cause of IBS

Megan, a 24-year-old recent college graduate, was planning a trip to Costa Rica with her family. During college, she had food poisoning and developed SIBO, and struggled with the symptoms for a number of months. *"I took the antibiotic rifaximin, went on a low-fermentation diet and felt that 80 to 90 percent of my symptoms had resolved,"* said Megan. *"I wanted to go to Costa Rica with my family, but we had planned a long bus trip to a volcano. I was terrified of getting food poisoning again because of what had happened the first time I had it."*

Her doctors suggested that Megan could go on the trip as long as she took preventive precautions and a half dose of an antibiotic every day to prevent a food poisoning episode. *"There were 20 people on the bus, and everyone got diarrhea but me. I may have been the sickest person on the bus because of my previous SIBO, but I was the healthiest person on the trip because of the preventive measures I took,"* said Megan.

If you've battled a gastrointestinal infection, you know it's not pleasant. Typically, the symptoms—nausea, vomiting, and diarrhea—don't last longer than a few days, but in some cases, the post-infection effects linger for weeks, months, or even years. The misery of a foodborne illness may not end when the acute symptoms stop. For some people, like Megan, that may be the beginning of months or even years of suffering.

Our intent is not to restrict you from traveling or suggest you stop eating in restaurants. Our treatments, including antibiotics and a low-fermentation diet, allow you to eat at any restaurant. You can maintain your lifestyle by using our strategies. You can stay well and live your best life!

Food poisoning, as well as certain types of infections, may precipitate a condition known as post-infectious IBS that occurs after an episode of food poisoning or parasite infection. Researchers have documented this phenomenon by examining patients with known cases of food poisoning, also known as acute gastroenteritis or acute infectious diarrhea. Whether the incriminating infection resolved by itself or with successful treatment, and stool samples indicated the infection was gone, certain patients subsequently developed IBS. This phenomenon has occurred again and again after sporadic cases of food poisoning or large-scale food poisoning epidemics.

We now know that one out of nine people who experience food poisoning go on to develop IBS. Food poisoning can introduce harmful pathogens into the microbiome and cause IBS, even many years later. It's also possible that many IBS cases may be secondary to food poisoning or parasitic infections. And while food poisoning is quite common, not all food poisoning cases later develop into IBS. Most cases of food poisoning resolve themselves in a week or two, without medical care.

When we ask our IBS patients if they've had a bout of food poisoning, not all of them can remember having one. Typically, we hear patients say, "I was on an international trip eight months ago and had diarrhea for a few days. Was it from the alcohol, food poisoning, or because I couldn't digest the unfamiliar food well?" When we ask our IBS patients if they remember what we call a "heralding event," most say they can't recall when the symptoms started. Others remember the date the symptoms began: they remember eating in a restaurant that resulted in food poisoning, and have suffered from IBS ever since. Many recall the diarrhea as the worst in their life and/or that they had blood in their stool or an equally dramatic event.

You may not recall a history of food poisoning, and you may not remember a few days of diarrhea. In fact, your IBS symptoms may have begun several months after the initial food poisoning. The constellation of these symptoms is called IBS, but its underlying cause is abnormal motility and SIBO up to 70 percent of the time. SIBO can be caused by other phenomena, but food poisoning is the most common path to SIBO. Anything that slows down or deregulates the gut causes SIBO. Food poisoning can cause the slowing of the small intestine and lead to SIBO.

The History and Evolution of Food Poisoning

When the first version of the Rome Criteria emerged in the 1990s, researchers began defining IBS for the first time. As discussed in Chapter 1, the challenge with the Rome Criteria was that IBS was traditionally defined as a diagnosis of exclusion. So, after you have a colonoscopy, computed tomography (CT scan), ultrasound, and stool and blood testing to rule out disorders such as Crohn's disease, ulcerative colitis, celiac disease, or colon cancer, your doctor can apply the Rome Criteria to ascertain whether you fit the diagnosis of IBS.

Around the time that the first Rome Criteria was published, European researchers found that people who were infected with *Salmonella* bacteria continued to have unusual bowel patterns that mimicked IBS for months afterward, and an examination of their intestines found nothing wrong. These patients met the criteria for food poisoning-induced IBS, providing the first clue that food poisoning could trigger IBS.

This finding was met with skepticism in the United States. Clinicians who believed that IBS was primarily a psychological condition related to a post-stress disease or anxiety disorder suggested that the finding was uncommon and may not indicate IBS. They hypothesized that food poisoning had temporarily damaged the gastrointestinal tract and that the damage could take a long time to heal.

But more and more studies showed that people with a history of food poisoning had bowel dysfunction that looked like IBS. As the data began to accumulate, the Rome Criteria committees began to acknowledge its significance, leading them to craft new terminology that identified this phenomenon as *post-infectious IBS*. It was considered a minor subset of IBS, but at least post-infectious IBS was now a recognized diagnosis.

For more than a decade, through 2010, post-infectious IBS was considered interesting, but only a small minority of IBS patients had food poisoning as the initiating event, and the contribution of post-infectious IBS to overall IBS continued to be minimized.

Post-Infectious IBS and Other Diseases

The first description of post-infectious IBS appeared in the 1918 book, *Medical Diseases of War* by Sir Arthur Hearst. He describes post-infectious IBS in soldiers with dysentery who developed alternating attacks of constipation and diarrhea after the bacteria had "died out." Developing a disease after an infection is not a new phenomenon and has been reported for decades in conditions other than IBS

Reactive Arthritis. This painful form of inflammatory arthritis occurs in reaction to an infection by certain bacteria. Most often, these bacteria are in the bowel (*Campylobacter, Salmonella, Shigella and Yersinia*) or genitals (*Chlamydia trachomatis*). Even after the infection clears, joints swell and lead to significant pain that can last for months or even years. Even though the bacteria had long ago exited the body, these patients show elevated markers for inflammation. A proportion of patients recover spontaneously, similarly to those with post-infectious IBS.

Post-Infectious Guillain-Barré Syndrome. This condition often begins with tingling and weakness that begins in the feet and legs and spreads to the upper body and arms. The symptoms are often preceded by an infectious illness, such as a respiratory infection or the stomach flu. As Guillain-Barré syndrome progresses, muscle weakness can evolve into paralysis. Nerves in the extremities start to fail, and the nerve failure creeps up toward the trunk. It can progress such that the patient can't walk or breathe because it affects breathing muscles like the diaphragm.

Post-Infectious Gastroparesis. This illness, which leads to persistent vomiting and weight loss, is acute and usually self-limiting. After the infection abates, the stomach is not able to empty completely or it takes longer than usual to empty. As more food accumulates in the stomach, symptoms of bloating, nausea, and vomiting occur. These conditions may resolve after a few months, but some patients suffer lifelong gastroparesis.

Post-Infectious Dyspepsia. This hard-to-delineate symptom causes a sensation of indigestion, usually after a bacterial infection. For example, an infection with *Salmonella* may cause diarrhea, and several months later lead to the development of IBS. Vomiting during the acute illness may become functional dyspepsia, which is a common but under-recognized syndrome comprised of bothersome symptoms that include a recurrent feeling of fullness after eating, the inability to eat a full meal or feeling full after only a small amount of food, or occurrences of heartburn, bloating, and gas.

As time passed, papers about the impact of post-infectious IBS began to proliferate. In 2017, Mayo Clinic researchers conducted a meta-analysis of 45 published food poisoning outbreaks, and found that 11 out of every 100 people who have food poisoning will develop IBS as result of bacterial gastroenteritis or infections with a virus or parasite.

We published a study modeled on the incidence of food poisoning data from the Centers for Disease Control and Prevention. When we overlaid the gastroenteritis rate in the US and studied what happened over time, we found that about 10 percent of those in the US developed IBS after a previous bout of gastroenteritis. This study, along with others, shows that food poisoning is likely one of the major causes of IBS.

Researchers have found that infections from a number of bacteria can cause IBS, including *Campylobacter*, *Salmonella*, and *Shigella*, as well as parasites such as *giardia* (Table 4.1). Some viruses have also been shown to lead to post-infectious IBS. *Campylobacter*, however, is the most common cause of bacterial food poisoning in the US and Canada. It also tends to make people sickest, and is therefore the most provocative bacteria for development of IBS.

Tips for Avoiding Food Poisoning

If you do get food poisoning with significant symptoms, it may be better to treat it right away with antibiotics like rifaximin for *E. coli* or other antibiotics for invasive pathogens. Of course, it's best to prevent food poisoning from happening in the first place. This is especially important if you already have IBS or SIBO.

IBS prevention with antibiotics hasn't been clinically studied, as such a study would require large numbers of patients in order to show statistical success. Furthermore, research funding for this phenomenon is lacking. That said, many doctors in Southern California—including us—take antibiotics to prevent IBS when traveling to countries at high risk for food-borne illness. As many as 50 percent of travelers to developing countries will contract some form of food-borne illness.

Table 4.1 Table of bacteria linked to IBS.

CATEGORY	MICROORGANISMS	EFFECT
Common causative bacteria that lead to IBS through food poisoning	• *Campylobacter jejuni* • *Salmonella* • *Shigella* • Pathogenic *E. coli*	Many of these contain CdtB toxin, which has been shown to lead to post-infectious IBS and SIBO in human and animal studies.
Small Intestinal Bacterial Overgrowth (SIBO)	• *E. coli* • *Klebsiella* • Possibly *Aeromonas*	These are seen to be elevated in SIBO and recently shown to predict a positive breath test. They can produce hydrogen in the small bowel.
Intestinal Methanogen Overgrowth (IMO)	• *Methanobrevibacter smithii*	These produce methane, which is associated with, and may cause, constipation and bloating. Called IMO since these may be increased in the colon as well as other parts of the gut.
Hydrogen sulfide producers	There are many including: • *Fusobacterium* • *Desulfovibrio* • *Bilophila*	These make hydrogen sulfide from hydrogen. Hydrogen sulfide is associated with diarrhea.

To minimize your risk of food poisoning, follow these tips:

- Avoid eating raw foods, such as salads (especially at a salad bar) or raw fish, including sushi.

- Always heat your food thoroughly. Don't eat foods that are left at room temperature for a prolonged amount of time.

- Avoid eating from street vendors or food trucks, whose sanitation is usually different from that in a restaurant. Food may be unrefrigerated all day and thus be exposed to microorganisms that can cause food poisoning.

- Avoid eating uncooked vegetables as they are often sprayed or washed with local water. Cook the vegetables and serve them hot.

- Drink name-brand bottled water rather than tap water, and use bottled water to brush your teeth. If there is no bottled water available, add iodine tablets to the local water before drinking it. Avoid the use of ice cubes, which are likely made from local water.

- When you bathe or shower, avoid getting water in your mouth.

- Eat at restaurants that have a reputation for cleanliness and avoid those with code violations.

- If you eat poultry that's been frozen, be sure to thaw it fully before cooking it to avoid *Salmonella* and *Campylobacter* food poisoning. For the same reason, avoid eating raw eggs.

- At home, wash all fruits and vegetables thoroughly before eating. Use a non-toxic food detergent, which you may find at your local health food store.

- Peel the skins off fruit before eating.

- Wash or sanitize your hands before eating.

- In hotel rooms, use disposable cups instead of reusable glass or porcelain cups. In some hotels reusable cups are only rinsed rather than properly washed.

- If you plan to travel to an area that is high-risk for food poisoning, you may want to consider taking half of a rifaximin pill with every meal during your trip, although this is not an FDA-approved treatment.

If you're staying at a rental home or bed-and-breakfast, take further precautions:

- Clean the countertops.
- Clean all chopping boards, especially if they're made of wood. Use separate chopping boards for meat and vegetables.
- Wash all sponges in the dishwasher. Sponges are known to carry tons of bacteria.
- To keep food from spoiling quickly, make sure the refrigerator is working properly.
- Pay attention to expiration dates on the food you buy. Expired food is more likely to contain microorganisms that lead to food poisoning.

IBS and Autoimmunity

Carly, a professional poker player, age 28, traveled to Mexico City and got food poisoning. After the acute diarrhea and vomiting disappeared, she became bloated, had significant abdominal pain, and felt very full after eating only a few bites of food. "I went to a doctor in Mexico, who treated me with antibiotics and I felt better. But when I returned home, the symptoms returned with a vengeance and I had to be hospitalized. The doctors did a workup and performed multiple procedures, but they couldn't find anything physically wrong with me."

The doctors checked for two antibodies in the blood that can identify IBS. One antibody (anti-cytolethal distending toxin B [CdtB]) was positive, but the other (anti-vinculin) was negative. "They told me I had post-infectious IBS and SIBO, and treated me with the antibiotic rifaximin. I got better, but a few weeks later my symptoms—belly bloating and diarrhea—came back. The doctors rechecked my antibody levels and this time the anti-vinculin level was very high. The doctors told me that my body had slowly started to produce the anti-vinculin, and that the disease had evolved. I went on a low-fermentation diet and took a drug to help my stomach empty more quickly, plus rifaximin to help with my SIBO. Now I'm doing well."

"If I hadn't had the blood test, I might have had unnecessary tests or months of treatment," Carly continued. "I have a high-stress job, and I wouldn't want to take antidepressants that might affect my thinking. Checking the antibodies in my blood led to the diagnosis of post-infectious IBS with SIBO and proved exactly what had happened with me after the food poisoning."

As we noted above, diseases and symptoms can develop after an infection is completely gone. With IBS, autoimmunity can be part of this postinfectious disease. An autoimmune disease is best described as a condition in which the immune system mistakenly attacks healthy cells in the body. Autoimmune disease can affect any part of the body, such as muscles, joints, nerves, gut, and skin, triggering inflammation, which can lead to myriad signs and symptoms. This concept of autoimmunity in IBS also explains why IBS appears to be more common in women than men, because women are more prone to autoimmune diseases; almost all autoimmune diseases are more common in women than men. For example, more than 90 percent of patients with lupus or primary biliary cirrhosis are women.

Understanding the mechanism of post-infectious IBS means understanding how IBS and SIBO develop. We embarked on a scientific experiment to find out how and why food poisoning can lead to IBS and SIBO. We developed an animal model of post-infectious IBS and we infected rats with Campylobacter jejuni, which is the most common cause of food poisoning in the US and Canada. We compared a group of rats infected with Campylobacter to another group that were not infected with Campylobacter.

Three months after the Campylobacter infection was gone, the infected rats had unusual bowel patterns as well as an increase in white blood cells and bacterial overgrowth in the cells lining the rectum. This was the first study to show how rats infected with Campylobacter developed IBS and SIBO from one infection. We thus confirmed that Campylobacter is a major bacterial organism linked to IBS, giving us an animal model to study the cause of IBS.

In addition, we found that the nerves in the gut used to initiate cleaning waves were damaged or reduced in rats with bacterial overgrowth from Campylobacter. That is, the nerves important to preventing bacterial overgrowth were reduced in rats that had had a *Campylobacter* infection. So SIBO, as well as IBS, can be related to a previous infection.

How We Developed the IBS Blood Test

We began looking for the toxins found in bacteria that might cause this nerve damage. We knew that the bacteria *Campylobacter, E. coli, Salmonella,* and *Shigella* all cause IBS and all have different toxins. We looked for a toxin common to these bacteria and found cytolethal distending toxin (Cdt). Cdt protein has multiple components. In subsequent studies, we found that CdtB was the active protein toxin.

The development of this finding took almost a decade, but we knew CdtB had to be part of the IBS process. When CdtB entered the bloodstream it led to the production of antibodies against it. To our surprise, we found that the antibody to CdtB recognized one's own tissue and reacted with nerves in the rat's gut, even in the rats that had never had a *Campylobacter* infection. This was a surprising finding, but with further studies we found that CdtB looks similar to a native protein in our body called *vinculin*. This response occurred only to vinculin of a specific molecular weight. This "molecular mimicry" can fool our body to produce anti-vinculin antibodies.

Figure 4.1 The evolution of IBS from food poisoning.

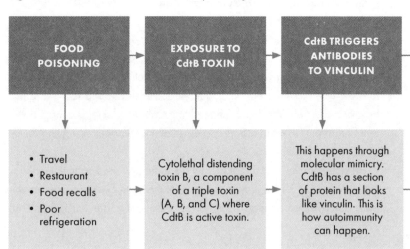

FOOD POISONING	EXPOSURE TO CdtB TOXIN	CdtB TRIGGERS ANTIBODIES TO VINCULIN
• Travel • Restaurant • Food recalls • Poor refrigeration	Cytolethal distending toxin B, a component of a triple toxin (A, B, and C) where CdtB is active toxin.	This happens through molecular mimicry. CdtB has a section of protein that looks like vinculin. This is how autoimmunity can happen.

Vinculin is an important protein in our body that ultimately helps the muscles of our gut contract efficiently. If there are antibodies attacking the vinculin in our body, gut function is impaired and ultimately leads to abnormal movements of gut, including the cleaning waves. This phenomenon can be further complicated by SIBO. By measuring the specific antibodies to CdtB and vinculin in the blood, we were able to diagnose IBS. This breakthrough led to the first blood test for IBS.

After multiple clinical studies to back up the data, we now know that food poisoning leads to anti-CdtB antibodies that deliver autoimmunity to vinculin. This leads to nerve damage of the gut, which slows down the small intestine's cleaning waves, resulting in bacterial overgrowth. These studies have further characterized how food poisoning causes IBS and SIBO.

The assay we developed searches for antibodies to CdtB, the toxin from bacteria-caused food poisoning such as *Escherichia coli* or *Campylobacter jejuni*. The presence of circulating anti-CdtB antibodies can diagnose IBS with diarrhea (IBS-D) or IBS with mixed diarrhea and constipation (IBS-M) that are linked to food poisoning. This reaction also generates antibodies to vinculin, and measurement of anti-vinculin antibodies further refines the test (Figure 4.1).

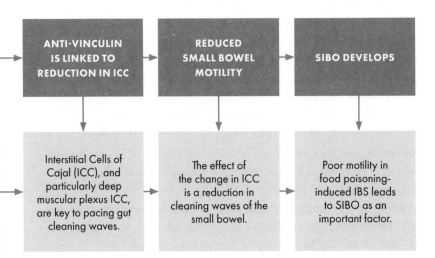

Figure 4.2 Change in antibodies over time in development of autoimmunity.

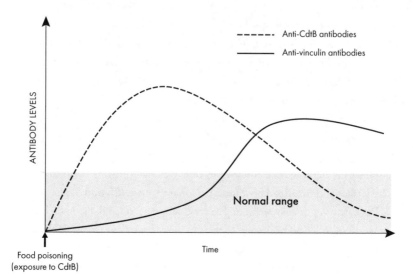

Based on a validation study of almost 3000 patients, we proved that we can diagnose IBS with greater than 90 percent certainty over other diarrheal diseases. If the test is positive, you know you have IBS, which is a real disease that can be caused by food poisoning.

It took us several years to develop the first version of this test to measure antibodies in the blood. Over time we developed an improved test that can diagnose IBS with 98 percent post-test probability, if both markers are positive (Figure 4.2).

Other researchers have unsuccessfully attempted to identify the biomarkers for IBS, but no other biomarkers have withstood the challenge of determining IBS positivity. Yet with this simple blood test, if you have diarrhea, we can confirm that you have IBS and that it's a disease. You'll know that your diarrhea is not due to Crohn's disease or ulcerative colitis with diarrhea or celiac disease. We can quickly ascertain whether IBS is the cause of a patient's diarrhea.

The test has limitations. It's not useful in identifying patients who have IBS with constipation. In addition, a negative test doesn't mean that you don't have IBS, as IBS may still be caused by other mechanisms. The test

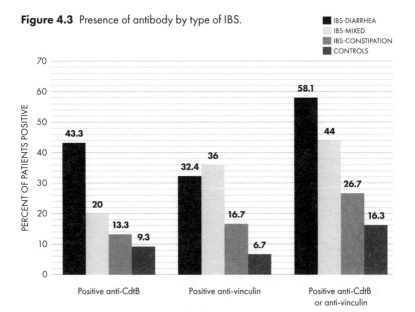

Figure 4.3 Presence of antibody by type of IBS.

was designed to diagnose specifically the subgroup of IBS that derives from food poisoning rather than other factors; however, up to 60 percent of those with IBS-D and IBS-M test positive (Figure 4.3).

IBS Blood Test Advantages

The IBS blood test prevents the need for multiple invasive investigations, and prevents wasted time and money to diagnose IBS. Doctors often order multiple procedures because they don't feel comfortable diagnosing IBS. Having a single test to determine whether or not you have IBS helps you and your doctor feel confident about the diagnosis. Based on past studies, it can take up to six years of doctor appointments and tests to reach a definitive diagnosis of IBS from the onset of symptoms. In contrast, this blood test takes only a few days to yield a diagnosis.

One noteworthy advantage of the test is that you can receive immediate treatment. If you complain to your doctor of IBS symptoms, you may undergo a colonoscopy, computed tomography scan, stool studies, tests for thyroid function and celiac disease, maybe even a blood panel to test for inflammatory bowel disease. These tests could cost $20,000 to $30,000, depending on how robust the tests are and how many times you have to visit the doctor before you receive an IBS diagnosis. Imagine the co-pay for this amount of testing and the indirect expenses incurred by you and your family members taking time off to go to the doctor's office for visits and procedures. The new blood test circumvents these issues. If the test is positive, you may be 98 percent certain you have IBS and you can quickly begin IBS treatment.

So one test determines whether or not you have IBS, thus stopping the madness of doctor shopping and myriad tests. And most importantly, it confirms that it's not all in your head; that you do, indeed, have a medical condition called IBS.

Summary

Because of the food poisoning connection, we now know more about the cause of IBS than we do about Crohn's disease or ulcerative colitis. IBS is 40 times more common than Crohn's disease or ulcerative colitis. We're much further along in understanding the true mechanism of IBS than that of the other two diseases. Yet in the last decade, Crohn's disease and ulcerative colitis have received $250 million for research funding from the National Institutes of Health, whereas IBS has received only $10 million.

Food poisoning was once believed to be independent of IBS, and now it has its own category (post-infectious IBS). Furthermore, we now know that many IBS and SIBO cases develop after food poisoning. We've found that more than half of IBS patients have had one or the other or both antibodies in their blood, meaning they've been exposed to food poisoning that caused the disease. Sometimes antibody tests are like road markers that read, "You had an infection," but the infection is not the cause of the disease. The markers of autoimmune antibodies show that the infection actually does cause the disease—in this case, IBS and in about 60 percent of patients, SIBO.

The next chapter examines SIBO and its symptoms and causes, and, most importantly, we'll introduce you to another simple diagnostic test.

CHAPTER 5

Small Intestinal Bacterial Overgrowth (SIBO)

J ennifer, a 30-year-old businesswoman, suffered from SIBO that had gone undiagnosed for several years. *"I had seen eight or nine doctors, and not one of them mentioned SIBO. I went to Cedars-Sinai and the doctors did a breath test, which was positive. Within a few days, they had identified my problem and started treating it,"* she said. *"It was so easy to define. When they told me it was SIBO, I thought how did this happen? Why couldn't this be the beginning of my story, not the end of it?"*

With all of her extensive investigations at many medical centers, Jennifer spent $20,000 in out-of-pocket costs. *"Other doctors told me to just live with it, or they would order yet another colonoscopy. It was frustrating. My medical bills started piling up."*

"Finally, my SIBO was treated with an antibiotic, rifaximin, and I went on a low-fermentation diet; now I'm doing very well. It's such a relief not to have to worry about planning a business dinner or locating a bathroom ahead of time just in case."

Introduction to SIBO

Many IBS patients like Jennifer have unrecognized SIBO, causing them to suffer through long periods of pain, bloating, and distension, along with the frustration of not having the appropriate treatment. Furthermore, they often incur high medical expenses.

Up to two-thirds of IBS patients have SIBO. The name of your disease might be IBS, but SIBO is more often its cause. Food poisoning is the most common path to SIBO, but as you'll discover in this chapter, a bowel blockage or any condition that slows down the gut can also cause SIBO. If you have IBS, it's more than likely that food poisoning causes the slowing of the small intestine transit, leading to SIBO.

SIBO is not unlike peptic ulcer disease. Peptic ulcers are open sores that develop on the inside lining of your stomach and the upper portion of your small intestine; the most common symptom is stomach pain. It took years of investigations for researchers to realize that an infection with a bacterium, *Helicobacter pylori*, was the main cause of stomach ulcers, rather than stress and/or spicy foods. Even after the discovery, many doctors didn't believe Dr. Barry Marshall's findings that *H. pylori* caused stomach ulcers. Dr. Marshall eventually won the Nobel Prize in medicine for discovering the association of peptic ulcer and *H. pylori*. If you test 100 patients with stomach ulcers for *H. pylori*, 70 percent of their ulcers test positive. Despite this knowledge, the name hasn't been changed to *H. pylori* disease; it continues to be called peptic ulcer disease.

The discovery of the relationship of IBS and SIBO took many years of experiments to show that 60 percent of IBS is due to SIBO. We haven't changed the name of IBS either, despite the fact that SIBO is the cause of IBS in 60 percent of cases. SIBO is not a primary disease in itself, rather, it's often the consequence of another condition. In the case of IBS, the condition is food poisoning, which causes antibodies that lead to neuropathy and subsequently to the symptoms of IBS. IBS is the disease; SIBO is the elevated cluster of organisms in the gut that cause symptoms defined as IBS.

What Is SIBO?

SIBO occurs when there are greater than 1000 bacteria per milliliter ($>10^3$/mL) in the small intestine. In SIBO, this excessive quantity of bacteria is not an infection, but rather an over-colonization of specific bacteria in an area where they don't belong. The bacteria aren't invading or attacking you; they are your own resident bacteria. SIBO is, in effect, a phenomenon of bacteria dislocated from your large intestine to your small intestine.

As the gut descends, the bacteria level varies. As we discussed in Chapter 2, your mouth contains millions of bacteria, but there are less than 100 bacteria per mL in your stomach. (We assume that the high acidity of the stomach kills many of the bacteria.) In the small intestine, the quantity of resident bacteria increases, but there are usually less than 1000 per mL.

The distribution of bacteria in the small intestine is unique in that its quantity changes from one end to the other. We showed in our recent REIMAGINE study that there are subtle, but very important changes in the types of bacteria in the various segments of the small intestine. In the REIMAGINE study we used a special catheter to sample segments of the small intestine while performing a specialized endoscopy (double-balloon enteroscopy) that's capable of reaching deep into the small intestine all the way to the ileum (the last part of the small intestine, almost 20 feet down). The most dramatic change in the microbiome actually occurs in the colon, which has an exponentially higher quantity of bacteria (billions of bacteria per mL).

The small intestine is an island of relative bacterial sterility between the mouth and the colon, which are filled with bacteria as mentioned above. The quantity of bacteria in the small intestine is somewhat controlled by the acidity of the stomach, but more importantly, by the transiting movement of the small intestine, the bile from the liver, and the digestive juices from the pancreas. This homeostasis is important. Remember, the small intestine is meant to help you digest food, not to "eat" your food, which is the consequence if you have too many bacteria.

The Origin of the Bacteria

Where do the bacteria in SIBO come from? While we have always believed that they come from the colon—which is chock-full of bacteria—new data may be changing that notion. The original hypothesis was that SIBO bacteria reflux up the gastrointestinal tract from the colon in search of food or nutrients. The *ileocecal valve*, which connects the small intestine to the colon, is a simple connector rather than a functioning sphincter. This means that the valve never fully closes and therefore bacteria can pass through it. The small intestine dumps these bacteria back into the colon when the housekeeper waves kick in, which occurs every 90 to 120 minutes during the fasting phase. (See Chapter 2, Figure 2.1.) When housekeeping waves are unhealthy and not frequent enough, excessive bacteria from the colon build up, resulting in SIBO and its symptoms.

The REIMAGINE study defines the normal bacteria in the small intestine as entirely different from the bacteria in the colon and the stool. With SIBO, there's an overabundance of bacteria with a propensity for higher proteobacteria (a type of gram-negative bacteria). Think of the small intestine as a lawn. If you don't mow the lawn (if there are no cleaning waves), the weeds (proteobacteria) that are always there outperform the grass (firmicutes, a type of gram-positive bacteria). In a recent publication, we showed that the two main "weeds" in SIBO are *E. coli* and *Klebsiella*. These bacteria are referred to as "disrupters." When they increase in quantity, they bully the other bacteria to die off and they dominate the small intestine with their presence and their effects. And, by the way, they are hydrogen producers, which we'll discuss when we address breath testing for SIBO.

In addition, the situation in your small intestine may be even more complicated. When SIBO starts, a war ensues among the bacteria in the small intestine, and the bacteria or microorganisms that win decide what type of symptoms you'll develop.

There are several subpopulations of microorganisms in SIBO, depending on which gas they produce after metabolizing food. One group of bacteria produces hydrogen, which can lead to bloating. Another group produces hydrogen sulfide, which usually leads to diarrhea, pain, and an urgent need to run to the bathroom. A third group of microorganisms is not bacteria, but rather archaea: single-celled organisms that produce methane. Methane affects normal movement in the gastrointestinal tract, and leads to spastic contractions that slow down propagation of contents through the bowel. That's why constipation is very common in this group of patients. We'll probably discover more microorganism subtypes, but these are the most well-known in SIBO patients as of now.

SIBO Symptoms

What causes SIBO symptoms? When food you've eaten makes its way into the small intestine to be absorbed, it's broken down into small pieces and then digested. If you have more bacteria than normal, the bacteria consume the food before you digest it. When the bacteria digest and ferment the food, they produce various gases: hydrogen, methane, hydrogen sulfide, and carbon dioxide.

The excessive amount of gas leads to inflation—like a balloon—of the small intestine. The small intestine, which mostly deals with liquids or solids, isn't equipped to deal with excess gas. When it fills with gas, it tries to move it forward. But unlike liquids or solids, gas can't be easily moved, and it becomes trapped in the small intestine. That's when you feel bloated and your belly may distend. You can't get rid of the gas because the small intestine is incapable of pushing it forward, whereas when you have gas in the stomach, it can be relieved by belching. Excessive gas in the colon is passed as flatulence.

There are, however, mechanisms for gas in the small intestine to disappear. Slowly, the gas is absorbed through your bowel wall into the blood circulation. When the blood passes through the lungs, gases are released and you breathe them out. That's why if you have SIBO, you often wake up with a flat belly because you haven't produced any gas overnight and the gas you have in your bowel has been absorbed into your circulation. Also, the housekeeper waves are active at night while you are fasting, and the waves push the remnants of food toward the colon, thus limiting the amount of food left for the microorganisms to ferment in the small intestine. When you start eating again in the morning, your symptoms return and become worse throughout the day. Generally, the symptoms such as bloating and distension are the worst in the evening.

The microorganisms in your body have been around for more than a billion years, and they have evolved to produce many types of chemicals and biologic substances, including lactate, pyruvate, sex hormones, histamine, neurotransmitters, and mediators that can directly affect us. For example, they can produce a form of lactate (D-lactate) that at very low levels leads to brain fog. We're in the process of identifying these neurotransmitters and mediators to better understand the set of symptoms in SIBO patients and, more importantly, how to target them in order to improve their symptoms.

The Causes of SIBO

STAGNATION

Bacteria don't build up magically without cause. Think of the colon as a swamp with slow-moving water and the small intestine as a fast-moving river. If you watch TV shows such as *Survivorman*, you know that a fast-moving stream usually produces clean, drinkable water, while a fetid swamp more often than not contains dirty water. Think of the small intestine as a fast-flowing stream, unlike the stagnation of the swamp-like colon.

Any factor that slows down the speed of flow through the small intestine has the potential to cause overgrowth. Such factors can include blockages—such as bowel obstruction—or any physical impediment, such as tumors, polyps, kinks, or adhesions in the small intestine from previous surgery. Motility issues can also slow down the gut or prevent speedy propulsion through the gut, which also leads to bacterial overgrowth. Sometimes motility can be impaired by a disease, such as scleroderma (a rare autoimmune condition), or by nerves and muscles that don't function properly, causing gut stagnation.

The most common cause of stagnation is a lack or impairment of cleaning waves in the gut, which occur every 90 to 120 minutes when you aren't eating. During the fasting state, these waves strip out debris in the gut after a meal. The salad you had for dinner last night has to be cleaned out so that your gastrointestinal tract is ready for breakfast in the morning.

Imagine that you turn on your dishwasher before you go to bed, but one of the cycles isn't working. When you open the dishwasher in the morning, you find food stuck on your cups and plates, which has allowed bacteria to grow on them. You pull the dishes out anyway and eat breakfast on them. This is, in effect, what happens if undigestible food is allowed to fester in your gut overnight. The undigested food just sits in your gut and can breed bacteria.

While the true epidemiology of SIBO is not yet known, the lack of cleaning waves appears to be very common. There are emerging data that suggest that damage to cleaning waves may be due to previous food poisoning and subsequent development of anti-vinculin and anti-CdtB antibodies, as we described in Chapter 4. Table 5.1 summarizes the potential causes of SIBO.

Table 5.1 Common causes of SIBO.

Inflammation of the small intestine	Crohn's disease, celiac disease, radiation enteritis (inflammation caused by radiotherapy for cancer)
Abdominal surgeries	Gastric bypass, any surgery with a blind loop of small bowel
Anatomical	Small bowel diverticulum
Medications	Narcotics, long-term use of anticholinergics
Autoimmune disease	Anti-vinculin/Anti-CdtB antibodies (post-infectious IBS), scleroderma, Sjögren's disease, lupus erythematosus, pernicious anemia (achlorhydria), mixed connective tissue disease
Lack of digestive enzymes	Chronic pancreatitis, cystic fibrosis
Lack of stomach acid	Achlorhydria, antacids (link is not yet clear; see text)
Endocrine disorders	Diabetes
Miscellaneous	Chronic intestinal pseudo-obstruction, intra-abdominal adhesions (commonly due to prior surgeries or endometriosis), mast cell activation syndrome, Ehlers-Danlos syndrome

GUT OBSTRUCTION

Anatomical obstructions in the gut, surgical complications, and certain diseases that affect the gut's motility can all cause SIBO. A prime example of an anatomical obstruction is a small intestine diverticulum, an outpouching of the small intestine. Part of the wall of the small intestine is weak, causing a pouch to bulge out beyond the muscle of the small intestine. The segment with the pouch doesn't move in sync with the rest of small intestine; rather, it stays stagnant and becomes a favorable environment for bacteria to grow. Unfortunately, this type of SIBO usually can't be treated easily, because the diverticulum acts as a persistent reservoir for reseeding the bacterial overgrowth.

WEIGHT-LOSS SURGERY

Bypass weight-loss surgery can also lead to SIBO. One-third of American adults are obese, so weight-loss surgery—or bariatric surgery—is more popular than ever. One of the most common types of weight-loss surgery is *Roux-en-Y*, known as gastric bypass. This non-reversible surgery works by decreasing the amount of food you can eat at one sitting and by reducing absorption of nutrients. Typically, the surgeon cuts across the top of your stomach and makes it into a pouch about the size of a walnut, drastically reducing the amount of food you can hold in your stomach. The surgeon then cuts a loop of the small intestine and sews it directly onto the pouch. Food bypasses most of your stomach and the first section of your small intestine, thus entering directly into the middle part of your small intestine.

This loop of bypassed small intestine is blind to food or liquid passing through it. Because nothing flows through those three feet of the small intestine, they can become stagnant. There are no effective cleansing waves flowing through it, however, bacteria can still grow—or overgrow—in it, leading to SIBO.

ADHESIONS

Complications from surgery or radiation, as well as tumors, can lead to the development of adhesions, or scarring, inside the abdomen, which can lead to SIBO. Normally, the intestines hang within the body's cavity, allowing them to be mobile. But bands of adhesions can prevent the intestines from moving as they normally do. And, as previously discussed, when the intestines don't move well, bacteria can build up, leading to SIBO. A prior abscess (a painful, swollen lump that's filled with pus) or a perforated appendix or gallbladder can also lead to adhesions, and subsequently to SIBO.

ENDOMETRIOSIS

This often-painful disorder occurs when tissue—the endometrium—that normally lines the inside of the uterus grows outside the uterus and may invade parts of the bowel and abdomen. The misplaced uterine tissue adheres to tissue around it and the body responds by developing scars around the adhesions. These adhesions can exist even without prior abdominal surgeries. The women we see with endometriosis often have adhesions of the abdomen, which affect the motility of the gut and lead to bacterial overgrowth.

INFLAMMATORY DISEASES

Inflammatory diseases, such as Crohn's disease and severe celiac disease, cause significant inflammation in the wall of the small intestine and inhibit bowel clearance. They can also lead to strictures (abnormal narrowing) that alter the gut as well and, again, lead to SIBO. This is particularly true in patients with Crohn's disease, who often continue to have a lot of gastro-intestinal symptoms despite good inflammation control. This is confounding for the patient and the physician, and may lead to an increase in the dosage of anti-inflammatory and immunosuppressive drugs, or even unnecessary surgeries. We have shown that about half of the patients with quiescent inflammatory bowel diseases with ongoing gastrointestinal symptoms suffer from SIBO.

DIABETES

Diabetes is one of the most common diseases that affect gut motility. This metabolic disorder causes your blood glucose (blood sugar) levels to be too high. One of the long-term consequences and the most common com-plication of diabetes is peripheral neuropathy, or nerve damage caused by chronically high blood sugar levels. This leads to numbness, loss of sen-sation, and sometimes pain in your feet, legs, or hands. The nerve damage can affect the nerves in the gut as well, leading to abnormal gut motility and subsequent SIBO.

AUTOIMMUNE DISEASES

Various autoimmune diseases can also cause poor gut motility. The most well recognized of these diseases is *scleroderma*. This rare disease causes thickening of the connective tissue, with symptoms including tightening of the skin, joint pain, exaggerated response to cold (Raynaud's phenomenon—when your fingertips turn white or blue when exposed to even a little cold), and heartburn. As the connective tissues become stiffer and stiffer, the skin gets tighter and tighter, thus disrupting blood flow through multiple organs, including the skin, lungs, and the entire gut. We recently showed in a publication that anti-vinculin antibodies are common in scleroderma as well. Perhaps IBS and scleroderma share the same mechanism of development, with scleroderma being an extreme form. In any case, once the gut is affected, a significant slowing of motility leads to SIBO. Another autoimmune disease, *lupus erythematosus*, as well as other connective tissue diseases, can also slow gut motility and promote bacterial overgrowth, although less commonly.

PSEUDO-OBSTRUCTION

Chronic intestinal pseudo-obstruction is a rare condition with symptoms that resemble those of a blockage—or obstruction—of the intestines. The symptoms may include abdominal swelling or bloating, abdominal pain, nausea, vomiting, constipation, and diarrhea, the same symptoms as SIBO. Gut motility can become so slow that it seems like there's an obstruction in the small intestine, but if a doctor looked inside the gastrointestinal tract, it would show no obvious blockages. The symptoms are due to nerve or muscle problems that affect the movement of food, fluid, and air through the small intestines. Once again, SIBO is common in this situation.

DRUGS

Narcotics can slow down the gut and lead to SIBO. The opioid crisis has led to many SIBO cases because narcotics precipitate bacterial overgrowth. The main effect of narcotics is pain relief, but they dramatically slow down the gut and cause classic constipation, as well as heartburn, gastric reflux, abdominal discomfort, and opioid-induced bowel dysfunction, which is a potentially debilitating side effect of chronic opioid use. Fortunately, we have drugs, such as methylnaltrexone, that can specifically negate the bad effects of narcotics on the gut without taking away the pain-killing effects.

Anticholinergics used in urology and gastroenterology to decrease symptoms of urinary infrequency or abdominal cramps work by slowing down the gut to alleviate cramps, which, in turn, affects gut motility.

Antacids used to neutralize stomach acid to reduce heartburn may decrease the amount of acid in the stomach, decreasing its efficacy in killing bacteria and potentially leading to more bacterial overgrowth. However, the link between acid-suppressing agents and SIBO is not yet clear. We have reported in a large study that stronger acid-suppressing medicines—called proton pump inhibitors—are not associated with bacterial overgrowth or any drastic change in the small intestine microbiome. Although proton pump inhibitors significantly affect the acidity of the stomach, they don't affect the acidity of the small intestine. If your small intestine is healthy, it can balance the effects of proton pump inhibitors without an overgrowth of bacteria.

We'll discuss a handful of other rare diseases associated with SIBO in Chapter 9. Although they are rare diseases, patients who have them suffer immensely. We hope this book will lead to dramatic changes in the recognition of these diseases.

Diagnosing SIBO

The all-too-familiar clinical symptoms of IBS raise the suspicion that you may have SIBO. Food poisoning is a precursor that raises the most suspicion. The good news is, we can easily diagnose SIBO with a breath test or bacterial culturing.

The primary—and easiest—method of diagnosing SIBO is through a breath test. Gut bacteria can produce carbon dioxide as a fermentation product, just like the bubbles in beer. We humans also produce carbon dioxide, so looking for this gas won't reveal whether the carbon dioxide is made by bacteria or by us. Bacteria and other microorganisms also produce hydrogen and methane, which is unique to them. When we find these gases in the breath, we know they come exclusively from microorganisms in the gut that have migrated to the breath. See Figure 5.1.

Figure 5.1a Normal lactulose breath test.

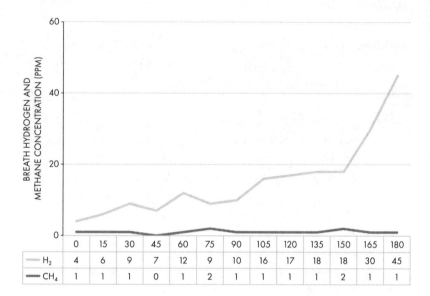

	0	15	30	45	60	75	90	105	120	135	150	165	180
H_2	4	6	9	7	12	9	10	16	17	18	18	30	45
CH_4	1	1	1	0	1	2	1	1	1	1	2	1	1

Figure 5.1b Small Intestinal Bacterial Overgrowth (SIBO).

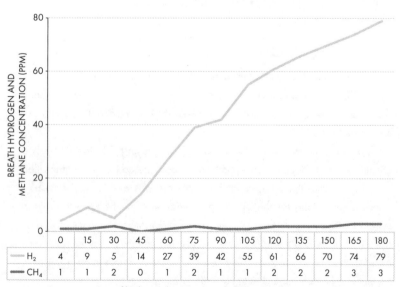

	0	15	30	45	60	75	90	105	120	135	150	165	180
H_2	4	9	5	14	27	39	42	55	61	66	70	74	79
CH_4	1	1	2	0	1	2	1	1	2	2	2	3	3

Positive test: Rise of hydrogen by 20 ppm within 90 minutes.

Figure 5.1c Intestinal Methanogen Overgrowth (IMO).

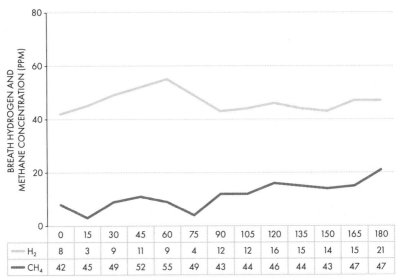

	0	15	30	45	60	75	90	105	120	135	150	165	180
H₂	8	3	9	11	9	4	12	12	16	15	14	15	21
CH₄	42	45	49	52	55	49	43	44	46	44	43	47	47

Positive test: Methane level ≥10 ppm.

Figure 5.1d Hydrogen-predominant SIBO and Intestinal Methanogen Overgrowth (IMO).

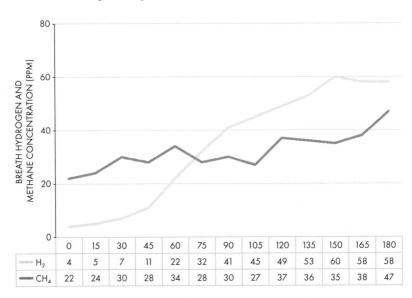

	0	15	30	45	60	75	90	105	120	135	150	165	180
H₂	4	5	7	11	22	32	41	45	49	53	60	58	58
CH₄	22	24	30	28	34	28	30	27	37	36	35	38	47

Figure 5.1e Elevated baseline hydrogen.

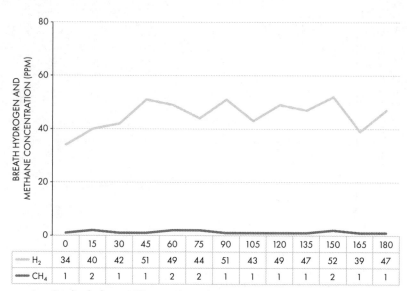

	0	15	30	45	60	75	90	105	120	135	150	165	180
H₂	34	40	42	51	49	44	51	43	49	47	52	39	47
CH₄	1	2	1	1	2	2	1	1	1	1	2	1	1

Baseline hydrogen >20 ppm without subsequent rise.

Figure 5.1f Flatline pattern.

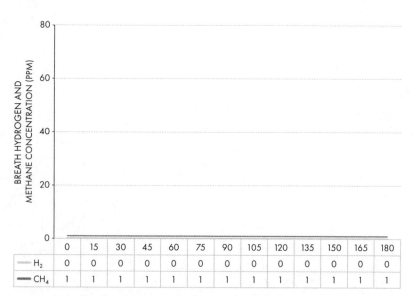

	0	15	30	45	60	75	90	105	120	135	150	165	180
H₂	0	0	0	0	0	0	0	0	0	0	0	0	0
CH₄	1	1	1	1	1	1	1	1	1	1	1	1	1

Lack of significant production of hydrogen and methane.

Figure 5.1g Normal exhaled hydrogen sulfide.

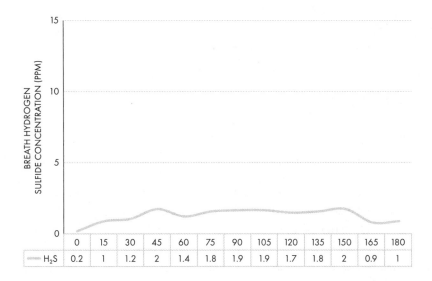

	0	15	30	45	60	75	90	105	120	135	150	165	180
H₂S	0.2	1	1.2	2	1.4	1.8	1.9	1.9	1.7	1.8	2	0.9	1

Figure 5.1h Hydrogen sulfide bacterial overgrowth.

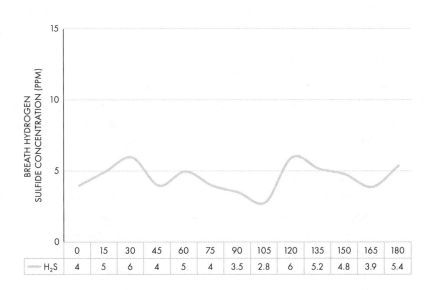

	0	15	30	45	60	75	90	105	120	135	150	165	180
H₂S	4	5	6	4	5	4	3.5	2.8	6	5.2	4.8	3.9	5.4

PREPARING FOR THE BREATH TEST

To prepare for the test, on the day before the test you may eat *only* the food and drink listed below.

- Eggs with seasoning (olive oil or vegetable oil, but no butter)
- Chicken, fish, beef, or pork with seasoning
- White rice
- Any kind of potato
- Water
- Coffee with no dairy

Following this bland diet on the day before the test will ensure that residual food in your GI tract doesn't produce gas during breath testing.

Eight to twelve hours before the test, do not eat anything. You may drink water and brush your teeth, but do not drink any other kind of liquid. Do not smoke, chew gum, or use breath mints. You can take your antacid pill and other medicines with small sips of water at least two hours before the test.

Be sure to check with your doctor if you have health issues that require you to eat special foods or take medicine for diabetes, constipation, loose stools, or for passing stool.

If you've had a colonoscopy or been treated with antibiotics, it is advised that you wait 30 days before doing a breath test.

BREATH TEST DETAILS

Hydrogen During the breath test, you'll be asked to give a baseline breath sample and then ingest a sugar substance such as lactulose or glucose. Subsequent breath samples taken every 15 minutes determine if the sugar has been adequately digested by you or by microorganisms in your gut. We use the sugar lactulose, which is different from lactose, the sugar found in milk and other dairy products. Lactulose is a non-absorbed sugar; that is, you don't absorb it into the blood stream. Because you can't digest lactulose, all of it is available for bacterial digestion. When the lactulose reaches the colon, which has a huge amount of bacteria, we may see a large spike of hydrogen in your breath. This indicates that a late rise in hydrogen after 90 minutes is due to fermentation in the colon. If the small intestine is extraordinarily fast, it's possible for the fermentation in the colon to start before the 90-minute mark, but that is uncommon.

Some doctors use glucose for the breath test; however, glucose is very easy for humans to digest. Most sugary foods contain sucrose— commonly known as table sugar—which is a combination of glucose and fructose. The body is designed to absorb glucose in the first few feet of the small intestine, but it's absorbed so fast that any bacteria below four feet in the small intestine won't receive any glucose. If you have bacterial overgrowth below those four feet of small intestine (which, remember, is 20 feet long), we won't be able to assess three-quarters of the small intestine using glucose in the breath test. Hence, we believe lactulose is a better substrate for breath testing. Lactose or sucrose can be used in a breath test for lactose or sucrose intolerance, but not to test for SIBO. Similarly, fructose testing is also used in a breath test to deter- mine if you have fructose intolerance, but not SIBO.

Over a two- to three-hour period, we carefully monitor your breath's concentration of hydrogen and methane. We wait that long because it takes 90 to 105 minutes for sugar to reach the colon. If your hydrogen levels rise by 20 parts per million (ppm) or more before or at 90 minutes, then we consider this gas derives from excess bacteria in the small intes- tine. If your breath test shows you are positive for hydrogen, then we have a confirmed diagnosis of SIBO. We have shown that the 90-minute cut- off correlates directly with the small bowel microbiome and also the gas production pathways of small bowel bacteria.

Methane We measure the methane levels in the breath at the same time as the hydrogen levels, testing every 15 minutes to analyze your breath sample. If at any point over two hours your methane level exceeds 10 ppm, this is considered positive for methane and you are diagnosed with what is now called *intestinal methanogen overgrowth (IMO)*.

Methane production is slightly more complicated than hydrogen production. When sugar enters the small intestine, hydrogen-producing bacteria use it to make hydrogen. This likely occurs due to bacterial dis- rupters such as the *E. coli* and *Klebsiella* mentioned earlier. The hydrogen is passed to methane-producing microorganisms, which in turn use it to make methane. We've identified the main culprit for methane production as *Methanobrevibacter smithii* (*M. smithii* for short), which is not bacteria but rather archaea. This is a three-step process: sugar gets consumed by one bug, makes hydrogen that is passed along to another bug, and that second bug produces methane. When the methane level in your breath is greater than or equal to 10 ppm, you have enough methane bugs in your gut to be consistent with overgrowth symptoms such as bloating and constipation.

Hydrogen Sulfide A test for this third gas in the gut is now available, and we believe it's a game changer in breath testing. Hydrogen sulfide is characterized by its rotten egg smell. This is unlike hydrogen and methane, which are odorless. Some bacteria produce excessive hydrogen sulfide, whereas humans produce only tiny amounts of this gas. Hydrogen sulfide production is associated with diarrhea, abdominal pain, and rectal urgency due to the overgrowth of sulfate-reducing organisms. In a three-step process similar to the methane-testing process, hydrogen made by one bug is given to sulfate-reducing organisms, which then produce hydrogen sulfide.

We conducted a large-scale clinical trial that identified the presence of hydrogen sulfide in the gut among those who experience diarrhea. We can measure hydrogen sulfide using experimental devices, and there will likely be a device to test for it on the market soon.

Carbon Dioxide We measure the content of carbon dioxide in the exhaled breath test as well. This standardizes the quality of breath samples so that methane and hydrogen levels can be reliably compared. Carbon dioxide measurement is not for diagnosis of a specific gut bacteria.

Your SIBO symptoms depend on which bugs get to the hydrogen first. Think of the hydrogen sulfide—reducing bacteria as foxes and the methanogen-reducing microorganisms as wolves. They're both looking for prey—hydrogen molecules, in our example. So there are two predators and one prey. If the wolves (methane-producing microorganisms) win, you become constipated. If the foxes (hydrogen sulfide—reducing) win, then you develop diarrhea. The winner for the battle of hydrogen can determine what you experience.

Culturing Gut Samples

SIBO can also be diagnosed using laboratory techniques to culture juice from the contents of the small intestine, but this is a much more invasive procedure. You prepare for the test by fasting for 12 hours. The doctor puts you to sleep, and then snakes an endoscope through your esophagus into the small intestine to siphon out some juice. The entire procedure takes 15 to 20 minutes, after which the sample is sent to the laboratory where a technician cultures the bacteria and counts the number of bacterial colonies. If the number of cultured bacteria exceeds 1000 per mL from the small intestine sample, it confirms that you have SIBO.

This culturing technique gives you the quantity of bacteria and has been considered the gold standard of SIBO diagnosis. That said, it can't really be the ultimate gold standard, as laboratories have differing culture techniques; furthermore, not all bacteria are culturable. Aspirations are taken from only a few inches of the small intestine, which may not represent the whole small intestine. What if the bacterial overgrowth is five feet down in the small intestine, which is not within reach of regular endoscopes? This technique may miss bacterial overgrowth in the deeper sections of the small intestine.

Contamination may also be an issue. When the endoscope enters through the mouth, it can drag bacteria from the mouth and pass it through the throat into the upper respiratory tract and then push these bacteria all the way into the beginning of the small intestine. Furthermore, each endoscope has a suction channel, so by the time it gets to the small intestine the scope is full of secretions from the mouth and throat. Doctors may think they are aspirating the small intestine, but in reality they've collected contaminated bacteria from the aspirate.

As a note of caution, some centers who perform aspirations report very high amounts of bacteria in the early part of the small intestine. One study from Dr. Brian Lacy at Mayo Clinic showed that sampling the small bowel with conventional techniques has about 20 percent rate of contamination, which is quite undesirable for a diagnostic test. We never see those numbers in our aspirations because we use a special catheter with a sterile barrier tip, resulting in less contamination. In fact, we see about half the quantity of excessive bacteria in the aspirate than do other medical centers, meaning that about half of the aspirate labeled as positive for bacteria from other centers is actually contaminated. If you're going to pay for a culture from the small intestine, it's best to use a validated technique specifically for the small intestine, including use of the proper protected catheter, proper sample handling to dissolve the mucus surrounding the bacteria, and a specific bacterial quantitation methodology. You need to know the exact amount with serial dilutions (your doctor would know what this means).

When reporting the breath test results, we follow the North American Consensus for optimal use of breath testing. We know the results of breath testing correlate with treatment response as it is based on physiology and the diagnosis of bacterial overgrowth. Some medical tests purport to correlate with treatment, but we don't understand how they work. Other tests help diagnose a disease, but don't correlate with response to treatment and therefore treatment management can't be tailored. Few physiologic medical tests have been validated in diagnosis and correlate with treatment response. The breath test hits all three marks.

Now that you understand SIBO diagnosis, we'll discuss the three pillars of SIBO management in the next chapter.

CHAPTER 6

The Three Pillars of SIBO Management

T his seminal chapter describes how we manage SIBO. Some doctors, even gastroenterologists, continue to assert that SIBO is "all in your head, just relax or go on a vacation." Clinicians are now learning to recognize and treat SIBO after reading the last book about our research.

The first step in treating SIBO is to understand that SIBO is not a primary disease; in fact, SIBO is a secondary phenomenon that's caused by other diseases. You may have a motility disorder that's causing SIBO. Or you have adhesions that are partially blocking the bowel, leading to SIBO. You are on narcotics for back pain and the consequent slowing of your gut is causing SIBO. Understanding the basic principle that SIBO is a phenomenon from a separate root cause will help you answer questions like "Why is my SIBO coming back so soon?" and "Why did the doctor give me a prokinetic (a drug to make the gut move)?"

Based on the fundamental truth that SIBO is not a disease, we break down treatment of SIBO into three pillars:

Pillar 1. Identify the cause of SIBO

Pillar 2. Treat the SIBO

Pillar 3. Use techniques (diet, drugs, and others) to maintain control or prevent recurrence of SIBO

Identifying Modifiable SIBO Causes

Identifying a modifiable cause of SIBO is the first important step. Identification doesn't usually involve expensive invasive testing; most causes can be identified by taking a robust patient history. For some patients, the cause of their SIBO is irreversible. For example, if SIBO is a result of gastric bypass surgery, the surgery can't be undone, so SIBO will continue to loom. Another example involves a small intestine diverticulum (an outpouching of the intestine) that accumulates bacteria, for which the treatment is challenging. We find that most cases are related to IBS and may be a consequence of previous food poisoning, which is now easy to rule out.

The first rule of SIBO management is for the doctor to identify, if possible, the underlying cause of your SIBO, and whether the underlying cause is modifiable. (See Table 6.1.) A classic example of a modifiable cause is a patient who use narcotics, which slow the gut and impair the microbiome, thus leading to SIBO. The most elegant way to address this is to help the patient stop taking opioids and restore their gut motility. While this is possible for some patients, others with chronic unrelenting pain (for example, those with cancer) may not have the option to cease using opioids. In this case, the best option is to counteract the effect of the narcotic on the gut. Fortunately, there are now FDA-approved drugs, such as methylnaltrexone, naloxegol, and naldemedine that can reverse the effect of narcotics in the gut without diminishing the pain-relieving effects of narcotics elsewhere in the body. Often the action of stopping narcotics or offsetting their action is enough to prevent SIBO relapse. Once bowel habits improve, the underlying cause of SIBO often resolves.

Inflammation of the small intestine due to celiac disease, Crohn's disease, mast cell disorders, and eosinophilic enteritis can lead to SIBO. In eosinophilic enteritis, certain white blood cells (eosinophils) infiltrate the gastrointestinal tract and also increase in the blood. The typical symptoms include nausea, vomiting, abdominal pain, and occasionally diarrhea. The infiltration of eosinophils causes a change in gut motility and stiffens the bowel wall.

CROHN'S DISEASE

With Crohn's disease, the inflammation stiffens the wall of the gut, leading to SIBO. In severe cases of Crohn's disease, the patient may have strictures, or narrowing of the intestinal channel. Treating SIBO in these circumstances requires medication to reduce inflammation and repair the bowel's movement.

A stricture is a narrowing of a section of the intestine that slows or blocks the movement of food through the area. Strictures are usually caused by recurrent inflammation. When the inflammation is uncontrolled, a stricture can eventually become a fistula. Fistulas connect two organs that are not supposed to be connected; for example, a channel may form between the small intestine and the colon or even the vagina. This situation is a recipe for SIBO.

The starting point for treating Crohn's strictures is to use anti-inflammatory drugs to reduce inflammation. In some cases, the strictures can be dilated using a balloon inserted during a colonoscopy or endoscopy. In other cases, the inflammatory strictures heal with a scar, which further narrows the bowel channel. In that case, you may need invasive surgery to correct them.

DIABETES

Diabetes is one of the most common human diseases, and the obesity epidemic has increased its occurrence. Diabetes alters gut motility, and when your blood sugar level is high, your brain thinks you have too much food in the stomach or that you're absorbing too much food. The brain doesn't know you have diabetes, so the brain slows the intestine down. In addition, long-standing, poorly controlled diabetes can cause neuropathy (reduced nerve function). This usually manifests as tingling, burning, and numbness of the legs. Diabetic neuropathy can also affect the gut. When this happens, the gut flow is impaired and can lead to SIBO. We find SIBO to be quite common in our patients who have long-standing diabetes. Diet management (Pillar 3) is very difficult in these patients. It is therefore vital to work with the patient's diabetes care team to better control the diabetes to reverse some of the neuropathy.

Table 6.1 Modifiable disease states that can lead to overgrowth, with diagnostic and treatment strategies.

DISEASE STATE	DIAGNOSIS
Narcotic-induced gut dysmotility	• Clinical history and temporal correlation of opioid use and symptoms • Urine toxicology screen
Small bowel dysmotility (post-infectious, scleroderma, pseudo-obstruction)	• Clinical history • Anti-CdtB and anti-vinculin antibodies • Bowel transit studies • Antroduodenal manometry
Intra-abdominal adhesions possibly due to abdominal surgeries or DeNovo (e.g., endometriosis, missed appendicitis, ruptured ovarian cyst)	• Sharp angulations of the bowel on small bowel barium follow-through (very hard to diagnose on CT scan or MRI) • Exploratory laparotomy/laparoscopy
Small bowel stricturing disease (Crohn's disease, NSAIDs,* radiation injury, and anastomotic stricture)	• Imaging studies • Wireless capsule endoscopy • Endoscopy
Active small bowel inflammation (e.g., Crohn's disease, celiac, autoimmune/eosinophilic/ radiation enteritis)	• Imaging studies • Wireless capsule endoscopy • Endoscopy
Small bowel diverticular disease	• Small bowel follow-through and imaging studies
Connective tissue disease (Hypermobile Ehlers-Danlos Syndrome, scleroderma, SLE*)	• Clinical history and physical examination • Visceroptosis (descent of bowels and abdominal organs in upright position) during small bowel follow-through
Diabetic enteropathy	• Clinical history • Transit studies
Dysautonomia (e.g., postural orthostatic tachycardia syndrome)	• Clinical history • Autonomic testing (e.g., tilt table test)
Mast cell activation syndrome	• Clinical history, abnormal mast cell biomarkers, abnormal number of mast cells on bowel biopsies

*SLE: systemic lupus erythematosus; NSAIDs: non-steroidal anti-inflammatory drugs

POTENTIAL TREATMENT

- Discontinuation of narcotics or switching to non-opioid medications
- Partial μ-receptor antagonists (methylnaltrexone, naldemedine, naloxegol)

- Promotility drugs (e.g., erythromycin, pyridostigmine, and prucalopride)

- Surgical lysis of adhesions
- Soft tissue mobilization with deep visceral massage

- Endoscopic dilatation
- Surgical repair
- Avoiding NSAIDs
- Treating active inflammation

- Anti-inflammatory drugs
- Strict gluten-free diet for celiac disease

- Promotility drugs
- Long-term low-dose antibiotic therapy
- Surgical intervention

- Promotility drugs
- Pelvic and core strengthening physiotherapy

- Promotility drugs
- Strict control of blood glucose levels

- Hydration
- Vasopressors and beta blockers
- Pyridostigmine

- Anti-histamines
- Cromolyn
- Mast cell stabilizer and modulating drugs

PANCREATIC INSUFFICIENCY

Pancreatic insufficiency or chronic pancreatitis can also lead to bacterial overgrowth. Pancreatic insufficiency occurs when the pancreas is inflamed or atrophied and doesn't produce enough enzymes to digest food well. With more food sitting in the small intestine, bacterial overgrowth increases. In these cases, pancreatic enzyme supplements can make a significant difference in helping the small intestine absorb food and keep bacterial overgrowth at bay.

DIET

We'll discuss diet a lot in the next two chapters, yet there's one important aspect of diet that's so important it's worth noting here. There are studies to suggest that eating beans can, in and of itself, cause SIBO. In animal studies, feeding rats kidney beans for even a few days can lead to SIBO. There are a number of possible mechanisms for this phenomenon, but the most important is that the carbohydrates in beans are not digestible by humans and other animals. As a result, the bacteria receive these calories and flourish in the small intestine. This is another cause of SIBO. While rare, this concept may have implications with other food products, such as overuse of sucralose, excessive lentil ingestion, hummus ingestion, and other products that are at times consumed in high quantities.

As our focus has been on food poisoning as a potential cause of SIBO and IBS, our understanding that IBS is related to an autoimmune reaction, and second-generation testing for anti-vinculin and anti-CdtB has helped many patients. Using the IBS blood test, we believe that elevated levels of anti-vinculin antibody predict the need for antibiotics and other medications to improve motility. In the clinic, we notice higher levels of this antibody, which means that it's unlikely the antibiotic rifaximin will be a one-and-done treatment. Perhaps you'll also need a drug to improve your gut motility. For example, if the anti-vinculin antibody knocks out your motility, you'll need drugs that promote motility. In some cases, we use the IBS blood test to justify the use of motility-promoting drugs early in your treatment.

In many cases, pinpointing a cause is not possible, and while we make every effort to do so, the cause is not always clear.

Decreasing the Problem Bacteria

The next step is to decrease the bacterial population in the small intestine to ameliorate the symptoms. In fact, this step can even be taken while the cause of SIBO is being investigated. Traditionally, we use antibiotics to accomplish the decrease, and we now have a microbiome-associated biomarker to tailor management: the breath test (see Chapter 5, Figure 5.1).

As described in previous chapters, the breath test can function as a treatment guide. If your breath test shows you have an excess of hydrogen without an excess of methane, there are several antibiotics to treat your SIBO. If constipation is your main symptom and the breath test shows methane production, the choice of antibiotics may be different.

The most studied antibiotic for IBS and SIBO is rifaximin. The advantage of rifaximin is that 99.6 percent stays in the gut and is not absorbed by the rest of the body. Other antibiotics also used to treat SIBO, including ampicillin/clavulanate, ciprofloxacin metronidazole, doxycycline, and neomycin may be effective, but they can be absorbed by the gut. Hence, they can cause systemic or gastrointestinal side effects, including allergic reactions and vaginal infections with *Candida*. When antibiotics are absorbed by the vaginal lining through the blood, yeast or *Candida* can take over. When antibiotics reduce a large number of bacteria in the colon, *Clostridioides difficile* can grow, producing debilitating diarrhea. Rifaximin has limited activity in the colon and doesn't appear to radically change the bacteria in the colon. It works primarily in the SIBO-infested small intestine, in part because it's soluble to the bile in the small intestine.

Rifaximin is FDA-approved for treating IBS with diarrhea. We believe the majority of IBS cases are due to a dysfunction in the gut's motility, which can lead to SIBO. However, rifaximin is approved on the premise that a subset of IBS with diarrhea is a microbiome condition. At the moment, the FDA has not approved a SIBO-specific drug.

In a clinical study called TARGET 3, approximately 44 percent of IBS with diarrhea patients responded to rifaximin treatment. More importantly, more than one-third of those who responded to rifaximin had no relapse nearly six months after treatment. This is a remarkable finding because it suggests that rifaximin impacted SIBO, a specific cause of IBS with diarrhea. A recent spinoff sub-study revealed that rifaximin was even more effective among IBS with diarrhea patients who had a positive breath test for SIBO (Figure 6.1). Other SIBO patients who took rifaximin showed improvement in symptoms without dietary changes, only to relapse.

Our practice is very similar to the TARGET 3 study. About one-third of our patients have a lasting benefit for months or even years after taking rifaximin. However, that is not the case for all our patients. Our IBS/SIBO patients who've had antibiotic treatments such as rifaximin fall into five categories:

1. **One and done.** You take rifaximin and, in effect, are mostly symptom-free for months or years. These cases require nothing in the follow-up period.

2. **One and better, relapse in time.** You take rifaximin, feel better, and then relapse within six months. In these cases, taking a prokinetic along with diet restructuring are helpful. While exact numbers are lacking, this generally accounts for about 70 percent of patients. Follow-up breath tests may reveal reasons for the relapse.

3. **Feel better, relapse quickly.** Antibiotics make you feel better at first, but within one month, symptoms return (sometimes within days). This is an important group and a second breath test is needed to test for SIBO. If you relapse and the second breath test is normal, there may be another reason for your symptoms. If the early-relapse breath test is positive, there's likely a secondary cause of SIBO, such as narcotic use, adhesions, or another structural cause. SIBO will return very quickly if there's mechanical reason for gut slowdown. In our opinion, this group warrants more investigation to rule out other causes.

4. **Partial response.** A partial response is also a conundrum. Could it be a secondary cause of SIBO? Maybe it's a placebo effect (you think you get a little better, but you're not sure)? Could it be that the medication was not taken properly? In any case, there are options to consider. In some cases, it could mean a second course of treatment, but other testing may be needed as well.

5. **No response.** If there's no improvement in symptoms, caution flags should go up, indicating further evaluation. The symptoms you have may have nothing to do with SIBO. There's a long list of potential causes for this, but some (while uncommon) can be sinister, like fluid in the abdomen or even cancer.

After exhausting all the different possibilities above, there's a very small group of patients who may end up on chronic antibiotics. Such patients have a significant cause of SIBO that's difficult to manage, but feel normal when taking an antibiotic. This is not an ideal situation, and effort should be made to avoid it if possible. That said, relief of symptoms in these rare cases might only be achieved with chronic use of antibiotics. There are other examples of this approach for selected conditions, such as hepatic encephalopathy (a condition where the liver is failing and bacterial products don't get filtered by the ailing liver, leading to mental confusion) and with IBD patients who have had surgery to create a pouch in the pelvis (called "pouchitis"). In less than five percent of our SIBO patients, use of antibiotics may be the only way to control bacterial overgrowth. Sometimes, we will alternate antibiotics. Either way, a physician's close supervision is necessary to monitor side effects if you are taking chronic antibiotics.

Figure 6.1 Response rate of IBS patients to rifaximin based on baseline breath test.

27%	26%	56%	77%
Average placebo response in IBS trials	Negative breath test prior to rifaximin	Positive breath test prior to rifaximin	Patients whose breath test normalized with rifaximin

Constipation IBS

Unfortunately, antibiotics don't work as well for IBS with constipation. As mentioned in previous chapters, a microbial link to constipation is the presence of methane-producing microorganisms (called methanogens). Methanogens are from the kingdom archaea; they are not bacteria. Antibiotics are designed to treat bacterial infections, not archaea or methanogens, although there is some effect that needs a special consideration.

But all is not lost. After studying the main archaeal methanogen, *Methanobrevibacter smithii*, we were able to determine that single antibiotics were not very effective in treating it. Treatment with rifaximin alone or with another antibiotic (neomycin) alone did not work well. However, in the laboratory, a combination of both antibiotics (rifaximin and neomycin) appeared more effective. As a result of this finding, we compared neomycin alone versus neomycin plus rifaximin in a double-blind study and found that nearly 80 percent of IBS patients taking both drugs felt better, and the methane-producing microorganisms were eradicated or diminished substantially based on methane breath measurements.

The result was a revelation. This combination is now used often in clinical practice. Note, that as a substitute, rifaximin plus metronidazole also works (although there is no published study showing this). Metronidazole would be a possible substitute for physicians if there was worry about side effects of neomycin for patients with kidney disease or hearing problems, for example.

The main challenge with antibiotics in the treatment of methane is that methane seems to relapse sooner and more often. In the double-blind study, constipation symptoms returned in one month in a large number of patients who initially responded to treatment. As a result, we have looked for other options.

As a final note, other plant-based "antibiotics" are also used for bacterial overgrowth, often by practitioners with experience or training in natural medicine. Some of these are worth mentioning, such as oil of oregano, neem, and garlic extract (allicin), but there are few publications on the efficacy of their use. One retrospective study suggested nearly half of IBS patients responded to these natural products. We are open to providing these plant-based antibiotics to our patients who don't want to take conventional antibiotics, however, the plant-based antibiotics haven't been assessed for their safety or potential interactions with other drugs. There are other questions as well, inasmuch as each product has a large number of options in the natural-product aisle of your pharmacy. Which producer has the most effective product? Which combination is best? For these answers you'll need to rely on those who have expertise in their use. Other natural products that may be useful for methane-induced constipation are introduced in Chapter 9.

Diarrhea and Hydrogen Sulfide

The newest kid on the block in breath testing is the measurement of hydrogen sulfide. A test recently made commercially available is the trio-smart® breath test that measures hydrogen, methane, carbon dioxide, and now hydrogen sulfide. The addition of hydrogen sulfide completes the breath test because these are all the main gases produced by gut bacteria during fermentation.

Adding hydrogen sulfide to breath testing was a significant feat. Hydrogen sulfide is a highly reactive gas, so collecting and transporting this gas was tricky. Secondly, traditional instruments have a problem handling moisture, so a new device had to be engineered for this test. In summary, the test needs a new bag collection system, a new testing device, and full clinical studies to determine the right cutoffs for abnormal. It took our group a number of years to devise this test (Figure 6.2).

It's important to know about all these gases. Earlier we described how these gases interact with each other. Let's go over this again. Even though measuring hydrogen predicts SIBO, we could never correlate hydrogen levels on breath testing with symptoms, even though it predicted response to rifaximin as described above. We now know that's because hydrogen is a gas fuel used by other bugs to make methane and now hydrogen sulfide. In fact, methanogens use four molecules of hydrogen to make one molecule of methane. So, if you have methane, it significantly decreases the amount of hydrogen you might see on a breath test.

Hydrogen sulfide is produced by sulfate-reducing bacteria that use five molecules of hydrogen to make one molecule of hydrogen sulfide. Hydrogen sulfide can now account for those breath tests wherein there seems to be no hydrogen at all (we used to call these flat-line breath tests). Many patients with flat-line breath tests had severe symptoms, so the breath test

Figure 6.2 How microbes interact in the production of different gases.

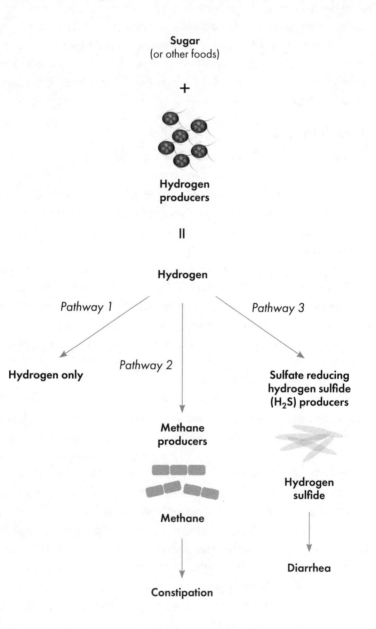

was unhelpful. It is therefore impossible to know the full profile of the SIBO breath test without testing all the gases discussed above.

More importantly, hydrogen sulfide is associated with diarrhea, abdominal pain, and urgency. In a recently presented study, we showed that, like methane, hydrogen sulfide is proportional. The more hydrogen sulfide seen on the breath test, the more diarrhea, pain, and urgency a patient is experiencing. That means hydrogen sulfide is really important.

How do you treat hydrogen sulfide? Since this new breath test has only recently been released, the experience with different treatments is still limited. What is well known is that bismuth can inhibit hydrogen sulfide production. Knowing this, our approach in clinic as of now is to use rifaximin (which reduces hydrogen, the fuel for hydrogen sulfide production) and bismuth (which reduces hydrogen sulfide production). This is likely to change as more data emerge in the coming months and years. Future studies will refine this approach, but we've already seen a tremendous benefit with this more complete approach to breath testing. See Figure 6.3.

Use of Statins

Even with the dual antibiotic approach, the methane-producing microorganisms tend to return over time. Since our patients who have IBS with constipation commonly suffer from this issue, we wanted a better way to treat this type of overgrowth. We learned through multiple experiments that lovastatin, one of the drugs known as *statins* that work by reducing the amount of cholesterol made by the liver, blocks an enzyme within the methane-producing microorganisms and reduces their methane production. So maybe we don't kill the bug, but rather block the enzyme it produces that helps produce methane.

It's interesting to note that statins are derived from red rice yeast. Red rice yeast likely produces statins to suppress competing methane-producing microbes in nature. In the laboratory, we found that various statins had different degrees of effect on methane-producing microorganisms. Lovastatin produced the optimum response in reducing methane. Our hope is that lovastatin affects the bugs, but not you. This is important because the side effects of statins include muscle aches, elevated liver enzymes, and interactions with other drugs. A recent attempt to develop a lovastatin that is non-absorbed was not successful, so this warrants further study.

Figure 6.3 How we handle patients.

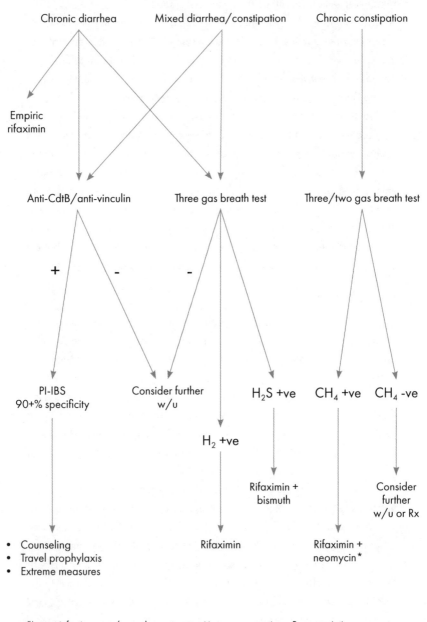

PI=post-infectious   w/u=workup   +ve=positive   -ve=negative   Rx=prescription
*Could substitute metronidazole

The Elemental Diet

Another more extreme method of treating SIBO is the elemental diet, which consists of a mixture of essential amino acids with non-essential amino acids, fat, and sugars. Often, water-soluble vitamins, fat-soluble vitamins, and electrolytes are also added. When choosing an elemental diet, it is important to choose one in which the daily allowance of vitamins and nutrients is 100 percent RDA-recommended. Our first published use of this technique used Vivonex® Plus; since then, other less formally studied alternatives have emerged.

The principle of the elemental diet is related to the ability to digest and absorb food. The faster you break down and assimilate or absorb food, the fewer calories or nutrients are available for the microbiomes in the small intestine and colon. The three main components of the food you eat are fat, carbohydrates, and protein. During digestion, enzymes break these components into smaller pieces, yielding fatty acids, triglycerides, monosaccharides, and amino acids. An elemental diet contains the broken-down components packed together; you don't need enzymes to digest or absorb them. The components of the elemental diet are absorbed in the first few feet of the small intestine. The rest of the small intestine is not exposed to nutrients, so bacteria are depleted of food sources and in essence, starve to death.

There is some evidence that an elemental diet may be useful in inducing remission in some SIBO patients. We most often prescribe an elemental diet if you can't tolerate antibiotics or have failed to respond to antibiotic treatment because the diet is very restrictive and can be costly. We've found that the elemental diet is an effective way of attacking SIBO. In our study published 15 years ago, a 14-day elemental diet was more than 80 percent effective in treating hydrogen-type SIBO. This study predates the use of and availability of drugs like rifaximin. Fifteen years ago, if you were on an elemental diet for 14 days you would have been more likely to get SIBO relief than if you took the antibiotics available at that time.

There are many challenges with the elemental diet. Many patients are unable to tolerate the taste of the elemental diet, even if the diet is flavored. If the diet is flavored, it's important to use flavoring that's not sweetened by sucralose or alcohol sugars. These are non-absorbed sugars that would feed the bacteria, thus defeating the purpose of your extraordinary effort.

Possible side effects of the diet include nausea and diarrhea. Also, because you have no source of food for bacteria—including healthy bacteria—prolonged use of the elemental diet can theoretically affect the stool microbiome, although the short-term consequence of this is unknown.

As with antibiotic therapy, if you have an adhesion your SIBO will return right after finishing your elemental diet. After the great effort to eat this liquid diet for two weeks, the return of SIBO would be very disappointing. As such, it's important to rule out modifiable secondary causes of SIBO before beginning an elemental diet. Although the cost varies, the diet can also be expensive, costing more than $1000 for two weeks, and it's generally not covered by insurance plans. It's not very palatable; our patients say it tastes "raw," and some of them can't tolerate it, even after adding flavor packs to make it more palatable.

Preparing an elemental diet is complex; it's not like mixing up a protein shake. Some companies produce what they claim to be a less-expensive elemental diet, but they've not been formally verified as a truly elemental diet, neither have they been studied in peer-reviewed clinical trials.

Prokinetic Drugs

Once you've successfully removed the imbalance in your microbiome or eliminated excessive bacteria, how do you maintain it? We know that SIBO can develop due to a motility problem and the lack of cleaning waves in the small intestine. There are drug therapies that can stimulate these cleaning waves, called prokinetic drugs, "pro" for promoting and "kinetic" for movement. That's exactly what they do—promote movement of the gastrointestinal tract.

Prokinetics are most often prescribed for constipation because they promote bowel movements. However, with SIBO what you really want are more cleaning waves. In our experience, using a prokinetic with food in the morning promotes bowel movements. But if you have SIBO you want more activity when you're not eating (when the cleaning waves happen). This indicates that it's better to take the prokinetic at night. Taking it at night ensures that it can clean the small intestine without promoting diarrhea. The main prokinetic drugs used for SIBO are low-dose erythromycin, tegaserod, and prucalopride.

Let's review gut motility again. Remember, you have two phases within the small intestine, one during eating, and the other during fasting. In the first phase (eating), after you eat the food, the stomach churns and mixes the food with digestive juices in order to digest it down to the basic nutrient level. The second phase involves rhythmic cleaning functions—those housekeeper waves of movement in the gut that move the undigestible food to the next part of the gut. We want to augment the second, non-eating function with prokinetic drugs.

Be aware that although there are several prokinetic drugs on the market, their use in bacterial overgrowth is off-label and therefore not approved by the FDA for this purpose. At this point, they are approved only for constipation. However, we published data that shows certain prokinetic drugs (tegaserod and erythromycin) do prevent SIBO, but the drug manufacturers have not applied to the FDA for this indication. Some insurance companies will pay for the use of prokinetic drugs for SIBO, but others will deny coverage.

Main Prokinetic Drugs

Several medications that we use can promote motility. They all activate receptors to activate motility and the housekeeper waves of the gut. See Table 6.2.

Table 6.2 Motility drugs by category.

PROKINETIC DRUG CLASS	EXAMPLES
Serotonin agonists	Prucalopride, tegaserod, cisapride
Motilin agonists	Erythromycin, azithromycin
Decrease acetylcholine reuptake (accentuating vagus nerve function)	Pyridostigmine
Somatostatin receptor agonist	Octreotide
Opioid receptor antagonist	Naltrexone

Agonist and antagonist mean activator and deactivator, respectively.

Erythromycin We use very small doses of this antibiotic as a prokinetic drug. In general, when this antibiotic is prescribed at 1000 to 2000 mg per day, the dose can cause nausea. Researchers found that a very low dose of erythromycin—between 50 to 100 mg at bedtime—triggers cleaning waves that can help prevent SIBO. We measure cleaning waves over six hours in a test called an *antroduodenal manometry*. A small, flexible tube is passed through your nose, down your esophagus and into your stomach and small intestine. When we administer a small dose of erythromycin intravenously during this test, we see cleaning waves within a few minutes.

At this very low dose, erythromycin has few drug interactions, unlike a higher dose. Doctors hesitate to use erythromycin as an antibiotic because higher doses can interfere with the metabolic pathways of certain drugs, such as statins. When used as a prokinetic, erythromycin should not affect the efficacy of most other drugs. If necessary, ask your pharmacist about potential interactions with other drugs you're taking before using erythromycin as a prokinetic.

Erythromycin is believed to be safe to use during pregnancy when used in consultation with an obstetrician-gynecologist. We don't encourage its use in pregnancy, but we've prescribed erythromycin to pregnant patients who suffer dramatically from SIBO symptoms under the guidance of their obstetrician.

Prucalopride This drug is known as a serotonin (5-HT4) receptor agonist that causes the gut to move quite efficiently. It acts on serotonin receptors in the intestine to promote gut movement and increase emptying of the stomach. If you take too much, it can lead to diarrhea. While no published data exist in the use of prucalopride for treatment of SIBO, it's believed to augment cleaning waves if taken during the fasting phase at night. If you take it in the morning, it can result in more aggressive bowel movements, so it's better to take it on an empty stomach at night.

Prucalopride is one of the most potent prokinetic drugs. If you take it after the bacteria have been eradicated, in our experience, the success rate is quite high in preventing SIBO recurrence. We performed a study in which we compared erythromycin to another serotonin agonist similar to prucalopride (tegaserod). The serotonin agonist kept bacteria away for over 200 days, while erythromycin kept bacteria away for only a few months. So, in this one study, serotonin receptor agonists were more effective at preventing the relapse of SIBO than erythromycin (but erythromycin was better than not taking anything at all).

One reason erythromycin appears to be inferior to prucalopride as a prokinetic drug is its short half-life, meaning it's quickly metabolized by the body. Prucalopride has a longer half-life and as a result spends a longer time in the body to allow it to affect good motility.

All of the abovementioned products have one issue that may reveal itself in time—a concept known as *tachyphylaxis*. This term is used when a drug loses its effectiveness over time (usually months). Erythromycin is known for this, but usually when it's used multiple times a day. The short half-life of erythromycin makes it less likely for tachyphlaxis to occur because by the end of the day most of the drug has been cleared from the body. The other drugs (prucalopride and tegaserod) seem to have this problem at times, at least in our experience. After a few months, prucalopride may lose some of its effectiveness to improve motility. To treat this, we put our patients on a "drug holiday" for two weeks, meaning they stop the drug completely. Once they resume taking prucalopride, the drug appears to work just as effectively as it did at first.

Why do symptoms recur even if you take prokinetic drugs? The simple answer is that there's no magic bullet for making the gut function normally again; the treatments are simply compensating for the problem. As a result, the bacteria of SIBO either return slowly or very quickly. We can help the small intestine become cleaner and stay cleaner for a while, but the SIBO will relapse in most people due to non-compliance with diet strategies and/ or poor compliance with prokinetic drugs.

Low-Dose Naltrexone This drug, which was developed to reverse narcotic overdose, is a partial antagonist of opioid receptors and appears to have other effects on the body. The opioid receptor agonists in our body can potentially slow down the gut, so low doses of naltrexone may help gut motility. Naltrexone is considered a potential prokinetic drug, but it's not as potent and its effects are not as dramatic as other prokinetic drugs. It's a safe drug for motility, but there are limited data on the true benefits in SIBO.

Further studies would be helpful to learn best how to use it. Other drugs that boost the vagus nerve (for example, pyridostigmine) or somatostatin have also been used to help motility, but data remain limited.

The Future

Twenty years ago, doctors would have told you that SIBO and IBS is all in your head, and might have prescribed antipsychotics or antidepressants. Now we have a greater understanding of the causes of SIBO, and as this chapter illustrates, our understanding continues to evolve and therapies are improving.

As we've shown in previous chapters, we now believe that formation of antibodies due to food poisoning is a significant event in the development of SIBO. A therapy that could eliminate these antibodies would be ideal and may mitigate the need for the other treatments mentioned in this chapter. Until we solve this problem, you may continue to struggle with SIBO even if you follow our approach of antibiotics, followed by prokinetic drugs and diet changes. SIBO is still a chronic disease.

While we've made a lot of progress, there's more work to do. At least, for now, we have some structured management based on what's really happening, as well as strategies to decrease the chance of recurrence of the symptoms of bacterial overgrowth.

Diet is another critical aspect of SIBO management, as we use diet to prevent the relapse of SIBO and IBS symptoms. The next chapter describes the history of diets for IBS and details some of the most commonly used diets.

CHAPTER 7

Low-Fermentation Eating and IBS

J amie, a 37-year-old school teacher, came to our clinic with typical complaints of long-term SIBO symptoms. *"I'm lactose intolerant,"* she said. *"I don't eat dairy because it makes me bloat. If I have dairy, I know it's going to be a bad day."*

While detailing her long medical history and many previous doctor visits, Jamie mentioned that even when she avoids dairy-containing products she still feels bloated most days. *"My doctor explained that I may have intolerance to dairy, but there's something more going on. If I don't have the enzyme to break down lactose and stop dairy, I shouldn't have any symptoms,"* said Jamie.

Most of the IBS and SIBO patients who come to our clinic have figured out on their own that they should avoid most dairy products, but often they are not just lactose intolerant; they have other food intolerances as well. Since most of our patients have a long history of gastrointestinal symptoms and have already had many medical work-ups, we don't usually see patients with isolated lactose intolerance. Such patients quickly discover that they can't tolerate dairy products. The patients we see who have lingering gastrointestinal issues may well have an enzyme deficiency that leads to lactose intolerance, but their continuing symptoms are likely due to IBS/SIBO.

There are a variety of dietary triggers that may have an impact on your gastrointestinal symptoms. In fact, up to two-thirds of IBS patients attribute their gastrointestinal symptoms to food. We focus our IBS and SIBO therapy on alleviating gastrointestinal symptoms with a combination of pharmaceutical and non-pharmaceutical treatments. The most traditional approach to IBS treatment prescribes medications such as bulking agents, anticholinergics, antispasmodics, and antidiarrheals. Unfortunately, this small menu of modestly effective treatments may not always be enough to alleviate your symptoms. An alternative, and more effective approach, is to manipulate your diet, by restricting certain foods that cause excess fermentation by your microbiome. This is especially true when using diet to prevent SIBO recurrence after treatments, as outlined in Chapter 6.

This chapter describes the most popular diets that have historically been used by IBS and SIBO patients, including lactose and fructose avoidance, gluten-free diet, and the widely used low-FODMAP diet. IBS patients have often tried more contemporary diets, including the Specific Carbohydrate Diet and the Paleo Diet.

Lactose Intolerance

Early diets for IBS patients were based on a simple admonition: Avoid eating certain sugars, specifically lactose and fructose. This advice was based on the observation of a correlation between intolerance to one of these sugars and the development of IBS symptoms. In fact, many IBS patients may not actually have a problem digesting lactose or fructose per se, but rather their lactose or fructose is fermented by gut bacteria before the small intestine has a chance to absorb them.

Types of Sugars Let's look at the structures of the three main simple sugars—glucose, fructose, and galactose. These simple sugars are called monosaccharides ("mono" meaning single, "saccharide" meaning sugar). Combinations of these monosaccharides result in disaccharides— two sugars joined together. For example, glucose plus galactose makes lactose. While bacteria easily consume disaccharides, they can't get readily absorbed by the small intestine without breaking them down into monosaccharides.

You need the enzyme lactase to break down the disaccharide lactose into its two separate monosaccharides, glucose and galactose. If you are lactase deficient, your body doesn't make enough of this enzyme to metabolize lactose. When lactase (the enzyme) is deficient, the lactose is malabsorbed by the small intestine. The unabsorbed lactose goes into the colon and is subsequently fermented by bacteria, producing gas such as hydrogen, carbon dioxide, methane, and hydrogen sulfide. The gas results in symptoms of lactose intolerance, which include bloating, abdominal distention and pain, and diarrhea.

Symptoms of Lactose Intolerance If you have lactose intolerance, within a few hours of drinking a glass of milk or eating ice cream or cheese, you may experience bloating, abdominal distention, and pain and diarrhea symptoms, as well as a feeling of fullness (satiety) and discomfort after eating (dyspepsia). When you avoid lactose-containing foods, the symptoms are relatively controlled. This is what scientists call a clear 1-to-1 relationship: one element is directly related to the other element.

Once you know the cause of the symptoms—lactose in certain foods— the simplest solution is to avoid those lactose-containing foods. This "avoidance of lactose-containing foods" became one of the first restrictive diets in the world of IBS. However, you may discover that certain foods low in lactose are okay to eat; for example, aged hard cheeses have less lactose. Parmesan and Asiago cheeses also tend to be less provocative. If you love cheese, you can probably eat the above-mentioned cheeses. You can read more about this in Chapter 9, where we describe our unique low-fermentation eating. Cow's milk and sheep's milk and their derivatives have the highest percentage of lactose, while goat's milk has less, but still significant amounts of, lactose.

You may recognize that the symptoms of lactose intolerance are similar to those of IBS. Studies show that IBS patients commonly report lactose intolerance-like symptoms, however, these symptoms are not predictive of true lactose malabsorption.

Causes of Lactose Deficiency So how does lactase deficiency happen? It can be genetic, but that is relatively rare. More often, after a bout of infectious gastroenteritis, the villi (small, finger-like projections that increase the surface area for absorption) in the small intestine are damaged because the epithelium (inner lining of the intestine) has been damaged by the infection. When the villi grow back, they don't necessarily produce the same quantity of enzymes, including lactase, that they once did.

All humans have a relative deficiency of the lactase enzyme. From an evolutionary standpoint, you don't necessarily need to drink another mammal's milk. In fact, we humans are the only mammals that do so. When most adults drink a large glass of milk, the full length of the small intestine is needed to absorb all of the lactose in the glass. The lactose lingers along the length of the small intestine as you absorb it. This is important because if you're lactose intolerant, it may not be because of a lactase deficiency. It takes the full length of the intestine to absorb lactose, and if you have bacterial overgrowth (SIBO), the bacteria in your small intestine may be consuming and fermenting the lactose, thus causing your symptoms.

Breath Testing One way we know that SIBO involves the symptoms of lactose intolerance is that we can diagnose lactose intolerance with breath testing, just as we can use breath testing to diagnose SIBO. If you drink a lactose drink before a breath test, we'll see a rise in gas production in your breath. This rise is not because your body didn't have the lactase to break down the lactose, but because bacteria in the small intestine fermented the lactose before you had a chance to digest it. When we treat SIBO patients successfully, about 30 to 40 percent of them who initially had a positive lactose intolerance test now have a negative lactose intolerance test, thus providing more proof of the involvement of SIBO in lactose intolerance.

We first proposed this concept—that the presence of bacterial overgrowth can lead to early fermentation—when we observed diarrhea-predominant IBS patients after a lactulose breath test and lactose intolerance test. First the patients had an initial lactulose breath test, and within seven days they returned for a lactose breath test and blood glucose measurement. We found a significant relationship between the hydrogen produced on both breath tests, suggesting that lactose breath testing among IBS patients may be a reflection of bacterial overgrowth rather than true lactose malabsorption. Doctors are now using breath testing to rule out SIBO before testing for lactose malabsorption.

Fructose Malabsorption

Just as with lactose intolerance, if you know you have fructose malabsorption, you may have already figured out how to avoid fructose. However, some symptoms may still remain, and this could be an indication that you also have SIBO. Unlike lactose, there's no enzyme to break down fructose. Known as fruit sugar, fructose can be absorbed but it's a slow process. After it's transported with glucose across the small intestine epithelium (mucosa) into the blood stream, it's metabolized by the liver. Fructose malabsorption, formerly called dietary fructose intolerance, occurs when cells on the surface of the intestines are not able to absorb fructose efficiently.

Fructose comes mostly from fruits, such as apples, pears, grapes, mango, and watermelon, and some vegetables, including sugar snap peas. It's also found in honey, agave nectar, and in many processed foods that contain added sugars. In fact, the consumption of fructose from high-fructose corn syrup increased more than 1000 percent from 1970 to 1990. This rise in consumption has likely led to an increase in fructose malabsorption and intolerance.

Eating a large amount of fructose can increase the water content of the small intestine and can alter the motility of the intestines. In addition, sugar alcohols, called polyols, naturally found in apples, pears, cauliflower, mushrooms, and snow peas, can also slow absorption and increase the water content along the length of the small intestine. If you experience digestive symptoms after consuming fructose, you may be affected by fructose malabsorption.

Fermentable carbohydrates composed of short chains of fructose with a single attached glucose unit are known as *fructans*. Fructan intolerance may coexist with fructose malabsorption or it may be the underlying cause of your symptoms. It's roughly the same principle as with fructose.

The cause of fructose malabsorption is similar to that of lactose intolerance in that the issue involves your body's ability to break down the bond between two sugars. Regular table sugar is a disaccharide combination of fructose and glucose. We humans have a transporter to move glucose across the mucosa, but we don't have a good transporter for fructose. Humans can't absorb fructose well unless it's combined with glucose. This process is called co-transportation.

A drink with a combination of fructose and glucose can be absorbed quickly. Interestingly, the food industry recognized the importance of this combination of fructose and glucose, leading to the development of a multitude of products containing high-fructose corn syrup, which has some glucose, but is predominantly composed of fructose. Today's market is inundated with sugary drinks that contain high amounts of fructose as the primary sweetener. Some of these drinks contain 50 grams of fructose in one serving, which far exceeds the human capacity to absorb fructose naturally. The fructose ends up in the colon and causes bloating, or bacteria in the gastrointestinal system find the fructose first and ferment it, again causing bloating. In contrast, humans can quickly absorb 50 grams of glucose within the first 15 feet of the small intestine without symptoms.

Even healthy people have trouble handling large amounts of fructose. In one study, healthy individuals were given either 25 grams or 50 grams of fructose. Almost everyone who received 50 grams of fructose had gastrointestinal symptoms. It appears that 25 grams of fructose is the cut-off amount that most healthy individuals can tolerate in one sitting without developing symptoms. To put this in perspective, there are 25 grams of fructose in a half-cup of raisins, two cups of apple juice/iced tea, or one 330 mL can of Coca-Cola. Your body has a low capacity to absorb fructose and can be overwhelmed with large amounts. If you eat two watermelons, no matter how good your gastrointestinal system is, you'll likely develop diarrhea.

Gluten-Free Diet

A gluten-free diet excludes the protein gluten, which is found in grains such as wheat, barley, rye, and a cross between wheat and rye called triticale. A gluten-free diet is essential for managing signs and symptoms of celiac disease and other medical conditions associated with gluten. This diet has also become popular among people without gluten-related medical conditions, including IBS and SIBO.

Celiac Disease A very small percentage of people develop an overt inflammatory reaction to gluten in their food. If you eat foods with gluten and feel pain right away, you need to avoid gluten-containing foods. Celiac disease is an immune disorder that triggers immune system activity that damages the lining of the small intestine. Over time, this damage prevents the absorption of nutrients from food—iron in particular—and you may become iron-deficient. From 0.5 to 1 percent of the population have celiac disease. Children with celiac disease can experience growth retardation, and adults may manifest joint pain and IBS-like symptoms of diarrhea, bloating, distention, and abdominal pain. If left untreated, celiac patients have a higher risk of bowel cancer.

People with gluten or wheat sensitivity (less than 5 percent of the population) also develop symptoms—abdominal bloating or distention, and sometimes diarrhea—after eating gluten-containing foods. If you have gluten or wheat sensitivity and you avoid gluten and wheat, you may feel some improvement in symptoms; however, simple avoidance of those foods may not completely resolve the symptoms. In this case, we don't know whether the symptoms are truly due to the gluten in the wheat. Studies show that wheat sensitivity has increased slightly over the past decade, but not to epidemic levels.

To diagnose celiac disease, we can perform a test to check for certain antibodies. We can also biopsy the small intestine to ascertain whether the villi have been damaged due to inflammation from gluten. Gluten or wheat sensitivity is not so easily diagnosed because there are no objective diagnostic criteria. We believe that SIBO plays a significant role in gluten or wheat sensitivity, as foods containing wheat are highly fermentable. If you have SIBO and eat wheat, you will have symptoms. Many of our SIBO patients think they are gluten-sensitive and go on a gluten-free diet, and they do feel better. When we remedy their SIBO, their intolerance to gluten and wheat goes away.

As with all sugar and carbohydrate intolerances, SIBO is often a contributing factor. Gluten sensitivity is a vague diagnosis, at best. If you go on a gluten-free diet and restrict your carbohydrates, you'll likely feel better. If you go on our low-carbohydrate, low-fermentation eating, you would also get better and you'd have fewer restrictions.

Low-FODMAP Diet

To improve upon diet therapy for IBS, researchers devised a comprehensive restriction of fructose, lactose, fructo-, and galacto-oligosaccharides (fructans, galactans), and polyols (sorbitol, mannitol, xylitol, and maltitol), termed fermentable oligo-, di-, monosaccharides, and polyols or "FODMAPs." When poorly absorbed, FODMAPs draw fluid into the small intestine, leading to symptoms of abdominal distention, and they also augment the passage of fluid and fermentable material into the colon.

As you know by now, rapid fermentation of carbohydrates by bacteria in the bowels results in increased gas production and distention. This leads to gut dysmotility and symptoms that can manifest as pain, cramping, and bloating. If you have IBS and consume high-FODMAP foods, a breath test would show that you produce higher levels of hydrogen than healthy volunteers. This suggests that FODMAPs induce increased intestinal fermentation and hydrogen production in people with IBS.

FODMAPs are naturally found in wheat, rye products, legumes, nuts, artichokes, onions, and garlic. As humans we lack enzymes to break down fructans and galacto-oligosaccharides. The more you eat of these foods, the greater the increase in fermentation and gas production. This leads to bloating, abdominal pain, and excessive flatulence.

The goal of the low-FODMAP diet is to restrict fermentable nutrients from ingested food, as reducing fermentable foods may reduce gas, distention, pain, and diarrhea in those with IBS with diarrhea. Over time, the concept of a low-FODMAP diet has been blended into the SIBO realm as well.

Studies exploring the effects of restricting FODMAPs in IBS patients have generally been positive, and they support overall improvements in gastrointestinal symptoms. Prior to the introduction of FODMAPs, it was not standard practice to restrict dietary fructans. Recent studies have confirmed the hypothesis that restricting dietary FODMAPs—in particular fructans and fructose—optimizes control of IBS symptoms.

Other studies have compared the effects of a reduced FODMAP diet to traditional dietary advice for IBS, such as avoiding larger meals and reducing fat intake as well as excessive fiber and gas-producing foods. These studies show that the severity of IBS symptoms was significantly reduced with both diets, with no significant difference in efficacy between the two diets.

The degree of malabsorption with FODMAPs differs with each person, so there's no "one-size-fits-all" approach. The general recommendation of a restricted FODMAP diet is to keep it short-term, initiating a full elimination for two to six weeks with the aid of a licensed dietitian. The American College of Gastroenterology recommends that you reintroduce a broad range of foods within one month of the diet. Your tolerance to a low-FODMAP diet may differ from someone else's, so it's important to tailor the diet to your particular needs and then gradually reintroduce foods containing FODMAPs back into your diet.

Please be aware that a low-FODMAP diet can change your micronutrient intake. Those on the diet may experience a decrease in retinol, thiamin, riboflavin, and calcium. Therefore, while a low-FODMAP diet may improve symptoms of abdominal bloating, gas, and diarrhea/constipation in IBS, you should avoid long-term use of the low-FODMAP diet in order to to avoid micronutrient deficiency. By the same token, a low-FODMAP diet won't protect you from getting IBS, so we strongly advise against using a low-FODMAP diet in order to decrease the chance of acquiring IBS or SIBO.

Over time, your microbiome may shift in a bad direction with the low-FODMAP diet. The microbiome of your stool becomes less diverse, and it's well recognized that having lower microbiome diversity is an unhealthy situation. If you're on a low-FODMAP diet for a long time, you may be malnourished and consequently your microbiome is malnourished as well.

The low-FODMAP diet is not easy to follow. If you decide to try it, don't do it on your own. You need to be under the care of a health-care professional or, preferably, a GI dietitian who understands the diet.

What's more, it's difficult to go on the low-FODMAP diet and lead a normal life. For example, one low-FODMAP diet app has 207 food ingredients to avoid. You can't eat vegetables or any butter. Mostly, you eat meat and rice. If you go to a restaurant, it will be challenging to find dishes that you can eat.

Other Specialized Diets

Two other specialized diets that IBS patients try, but have not been well studied, include the Specific Carbohydrate Diet and the Paleo Diet. They have a lot of similarities to other diets we've already mentioned.

SPECIFIC CARBOHYDRATE DIET

The Specific Carbohydrate Diet is a spinoff of the gluten-free diet. During this very detailed diet, you restrict complex carbohydrates and limit the sugars you eat to mostly monosaccharides. The gist is to eat fewer carbohydrates. Complex carbohydrates contain more fiber—thus, their potential for fermenting. The more complex the carbohydrate, the harder it is to digest, leaving it for the bacteria to digest and ferment, resulting in gas and gastrointestinal symptoms.

Like the low-FODMAP diet, the Specific Carbohydrate Diet is difficult to follow. It's very similar to the low-FODMAP diet, but it's not as commonly used for IBS patients. One clinical study compared the low-FODMAP diet to the Specific Carbohydrate Diet for IBS patients, and it was found that the low-FODMAP diet relieved symptoms but the Specific Carbohydrate Diet did not.

IBS patients don't necessarily do well on the Specific Carbohydrate Diet. It includes dairy products, such as yogurt and cheese, as well as dried fruit. Therefore, not many IBS or SIBO patients can tolerate the Specialized Carbohydrate Diet. Other patients, including those with Crohn's disease, colitis, celiac disease, and autism, may use the Specialized Carbohydrate Diet. There's no hard data to support its use in these disorders, but it has a large following nevertheless.

PALEO DIET

The Paleo Diet is easier to follow than the Specialized Carbohydrate Diet. This diet is based on foods similar to what we might have eaten during the Paleolithic era, which occurred approximately 2.5 million to 10,000 years ago. Its premise is based on the fact that early humans were cave-dwelling people who ate mostly berries and meat and very little carbohydrates. We weren't an agricultural society for millions of years, so our bodies were likely designed to eat this way.

A Paleo Diet typically includes lean meats, fish, fruits, vegetables, nuts, and seeds—foods that in the past could be obtained by hunting and gathering. The diet limits foods that became common when farming emerged, such as dairy products, legumes, and grains. There are many online resources, and most dietitians will know how to guide you.

The Paleo Diet was designed for weight loss and weight management, not specifically for SIBO management. Because it's low in carbohydrates, and therefore contains fewer fermentable foods, IBS patients may feel better at first because bacteria in the gut won't have enough material to ferment. This restrictive diet is potentially nutritionally deficient, specifically calcium deficient.

In summary, we like to tell our patients, "If you eat nothing, your IBS and SIBO will go away or get better." Obviously, this is a joke, but it emphasizes the point that you share your food with your bacteria. The more restrictive the diet, the more likely a SIBO patient will respond. You will have fewer calories for bacteria to ferment food, but also fewer calories for you, which is not healthy. Obviously, everyone has to eat to survive.

Diets like the low-FODMAP diet may confuse dietitians, let alone patients and doctors. The dietary advice now available online about the low-FODMAP diet can be contradictory. The Specialized Carbohydrate Diet and Paleo Diet were *not* designed for SIBO patients.

In the next chapter, we outline our detailed low-fermentation eating, which we designed specifically for SIBO patients. We provide simple but robust dietary advice on how to restrict certain foods, while including a veritable smorgasbord of foods that you can still eat, both at home and in restaurants.

CHAPTER 8

The Low-Fermentation Diet

In the early 2000s we began developing a diet plan for patients with SIBO called *low-fermentation eating*. Our ultimate goal was to develop a diet based on the rational science regarding IBS/SIBO, but more importantly, we wanted a diet that allowed patients to live as normal a life as possible. With low-fermentation eating, you should be able to travel, and you can go to a restaurant and find food you can eat on almost any menu. And you won't have to ask the server countless questions about what you're ordering.

We designed this diet with you in mind. You can be yourself instead of feeling burdened by the extremes of a restrictive diet; you don't have to avoid *everything* to receive the benefits of this diet. And low-fermentation eating was developed in collaboration with dietitians, so it's nutritionally balanced, making nutritional deficiencies far less likely.

The composition of the low-fermentation eating falls within the context of current scientific knowledge regarding the microbiome itself, the interaction of the human body with the microbiome and food, and the pathophysiology of IBS/SIBO. Low-fermentation eating is not just about *what* you eat, but also *when* you eat and how you space meals to allow for the cleaning waves that form the low-fermentation diet.

This chapter outlines the composition of low-fermentation eating and also introduces lifestyle changes, reviews the physiologic mechanism of digestion, and teaches you when to eat and when not to eat. Understanding these concepts may take some time, but once you learn them, you'll be better able to manage your situation.

Origins

Low-fermentation eating originates from our knowledge of microbes. If you leave a teaspoon of olive oil on the counter, bacteria won't grow on the oil. But if you mix a teaspoon of sugar (carbohydrate) into the oil, within a few days bacteria and fungi will ferment and spoil the oil. Carbohydrates are one of the main energy sources for bacteria, and when bacteria ferment carbohydrates, the sugar converts to gas that causes the bloating and abdominal distention of SIBO. The predominant driver of SIBO symptoms is sugar. Yes, we need sugar, but bacteria need sugar as well. If you can eliminate sugars that humans don't digest and limit your intake of fiber (which is difficult to digest) you can limit your SIBO symptoms and decrease the chance of recurrence of SIBO.

Low-Fermentation Eating

Low-fermentation eating has two essential rules:

1. Restrict products that contain high levels of carbohydrates or ingredients in food that humans can't digest, and therefore are digested by bacteria.

2. Space meals four to five hours apart.

FOODS TO AVOID

At the top of the list of foods to avoid are non-absorbable sugars, such as sucralose, sorbitol, lactitol, xylitol, and mannitol. Humans can't digest these artificial sweeteners, and therefore 100 percent of their calories are available for bacteria to digest. Non-digestible sugars will always cause bloating. For the same reason, you should avoid sugar-free gum, which often contains artificial sweeteners.

The good news is you can eat products that contain the artificial sweetener aspartame found in Equal. Aspartame is a peptide, not a sugar, which makes it both digestible and sweet tasting. If you like to chew gum, consider gums made with glucose, a completely absorbable sugar. Glee Gum and Simply Gum are examples.

Unfortunately, food manufacturers sneak non-absorbable sugars into food and often you won't know they're there. For example, many soft drinks once made with aspartame are now made with sucralose and often the label doesn't announce "new formulation." We discovered this when our IBS/SIBO patients began telling us that their bloating returned, despite maintaining their low-fermentation eating. You may not be aware that your favorite drink has switched sweeteners and may now be harmful to your gastrointestinal microbiome health if you have IBS or SIBO. It's very important to read food labels, looking specifically for sorbitol, sucralose, and other sugar alcohols that are non-absorbable.

Look for hidden inulin. *Inulin* is another food additive that may bother your gastrointestinal tract. Inulin is a type of fructan and prebiotic, a compound in food that can induce the growth or activity of micro-organisms, such as bacteria. It's extracted from chicory root fiber—a natural dietary fiber—and may also be found in smaller amounts in whole wheat and some vegetables and fruits, such as asparagus, garlic, and bananas. Inulin has a creamy mouth feel, so it's often used to help reduce the fat content in products. Because it tastes slightly sweet, it's also used to help reduce some of the sugar and sugar substitutes found in foods and beverages.

Like fiber, inulin can cause gas, bloating, and abdominal pain, particularly if you have IBS or SIBO. Chicory root fiber passes through your small intestine and is fermented by bacteria in your large intestine. People who are more sensitive to inulin may need to limit its consumption.

Inulin does, however, have some digestive benefits. It appears to help with constipation, and the fiber increases the amounts of beneficial *Bifidobacteria* and *Lactobacilli* bacteria in the gut.

Unfortunately, manufacturers are not required to specify the amount of inulin on their products' labels. Instead, you'll find inulin included in the total amount of dietary fiber on the Nutrition Facts table. If a food or beverage that doesn't usually contain fiber—such as yogurt or flavored water—lists inulin as the only fiber ingredient, the amount of dietary fiber tells you how many grams of inulin have been added.

If a food—such as a cereal or a granola bar—is made with whole grains or other fiber-rich ingredients, it can be difficult to tell how much of the fiber is coming from inulin. Look at the ingredients list to see where the inulin appears. It could be listed as inulin, oligofructose, oligofructose-enriched inulin, chicory root fiber, chicory root extract, or fructo-oligosaccharides. Ingredients are listed by weight, so if inulin shows up early in the list, higher amounts of it have been added. In general, the fewer ingredients on the label, the better off you are.

RESTRICT NON-DIGESTIBLE CARBOHYDRATE-CONTAINING FOODS

When you think of a non-digestible carbohydrate, think of fiber. Fiber is a carbohydrate that can't be broken down by the body. It either passes through the digestive system unchanged (insoluble fiber), or is fermented by intestinal bacteria in the colon (soluble fiber). Fiber is found in intact plant foods, including fruits, vegetables, legumes, nuts, seeds, and whole grains. It can also be isolated and added to processed foods and fiber supplements (see inulin, above).

In general, if you have IBS or SIBO, you'll need to limit or eliminate high-fiber foods. When we advise less fiber in your diet, it doesn't matter whether it's soluble or insoluble. Less fiber means less gas production in the small intestine. You'll need to eat fewer vegetables that have fiber, such as cruciferous vegetables, cabbage, sauerkraut, Brussels sprouts, and broccoli.

More importantly, take note of the simpler carbohydrates that are harder to digest. The simpler the carbohydrate, the faster they break down and assimilate in your gut. However, if humans can't break the chain of sugars in these simpler forms, they're used by bacteria that can quickly and easily break them down. This results in more rapid gas production and thus your uncomfortable symptoms of bloating and pain. We consider these foods as absolute "no-no's" because of how quickly and potently they can worsen symptoms in SIBO and IBS. Some carbohydrates to avoid include black beans, pinto beans, kidney beans, and lupini beans. Chickpeas (the primary ingredient in hummus) can be extremely provocative. Lentils are an important source of protein among vegans and in certain Asian cultures; however, when SIBO is present, these legumes are among the worst provocateurs.

Milk and other dairy products, such as yogurt and cheese, deserve special mention here, as it's well known that these can cause gas and bloating. Dairy products contain lactose sugar that is problematic. Humans can digest a certain amount of lactose; however, the amount varies from person to person, based on ethnic origin and age. As you age, you become less able to digest lactose. If you don't digest this very simple sugar, the bacteria of the gut surely will, and this produces gas. The food industry is well aware of this problem and has developed many lactose-free options for milk, ice cream, and other products. But beware: always check the ingredients. Lactose-free ice cream is fine to eat, but be on the lookout for added sucralose or inulin.

TIME YOUR EATING

Cleaning Waves We can't emphasize enough the importance of keeping the gastrointestinal tract's cleaning waves intact on a regular basis. These cleaning waves (as mentioned in previous chapters) keep the small bowel clean, and they reduce bacteria therein. Notably, the housekeeping waves don't occur until you are fasting. The feeding phase of digestion ends within one to four hours of eating, and then the housekeeping wave cycles begin. Based on this time frame, we recommend waiting four to five hours between each meal as part of low-fermentation eating. That will result in at least one set of housekeeping waves between each meal. This timing procedure will keep the small intestine clean of bacteria and residual foods, as well as residual enzymes that were secreted to move food through the gastrointestinal tract.

Patients with SIBO often have a reduced number of cleaning waves, so the fasting period between meals may not mean every gap produces a cleaning wave as it might in normal people. However, snacking between meals is a no-no. If you eat every two hours, you won't allow the small intestine to clear properly (even if you don't have SIBO or IBS), and food will pile up. This leads to an overgrowth of bacteria in the small intestine if your motility is not in good working order. Just one bite of food can impair your cleaning waves!

Meal Timing Overnight is the longest period of fasting for most people. As a result, your small intestine experiences the most cleaning waves and your body is able to clear out a greater number of bacteria. Eating before bed will shift the small intestine from "cleaning mode" to "eating mode" and as a result, there will be less time for bacteria to be cleared. Avoid eating close to bedtime, and don't get up in the middle of the night for a bite to eat. Eating even a small amount of food stops the cleaning function and triggers the switch to eating mode. If you wake up hungry at 3:00 A.M. and eat even a small amount of food, the small intestine's clock resets and thus throws off the cleaning wave cycle.

Let's take a quick look at human evolution. In North America inhabitants lived on the plains, killing and eating game such as buffalo, and eating roots and vegetables. There was no way to refrigerate food. You ate whatever you caught or gathered that day. This is the feast and famine environment from which we evolved. Early humans would eat a lot one day and then wouldn't eat for a day or two, until the next hunt and kill. Cleaning waves evolved to occur during fasting, so if you curtail them by constant eating, it creates an abnormal situation in your gut.

Snacking Snacking is new to human culture. It began in the 20th century with the invention of refrigeration, and is now very much part of our culture. Many workplaces now have kitchens and vending machines, and snacks are often placed all around the workplace. TV commercials show a person at work feeling tired and grabbing a candy bar to renew their energy. Snacking is not necessarily a healthy habit and it is decidedly worse for SIBO patients.

Beverages What about coffee or water in between meals? Generally, it's okay because beverages don't convert to a feeding state thereby creating cleaning waves. Between meals, we recommend black coffee, tea, or plain water.

Water is very important. While there's a current focus on drinking more water in general, too much water can also be harmful. Drinking adequate amounts of water will promote movement in the gastrointestinal tract and may help motility in the small intestine.

There are some myths to be aware of. Patients with constipation often drink many glasses of water a day to encourage bowel movements. This doesn't work! For example, we had a patient with severe constipation (only one bowel movement every two weeks). In an effort to help herself, she drank two to three gallons of water every day for a period of time. This practice severely reduced the sodium in her blood, sending her to the hospital.

Water is key to our survival. The human intestine will absorb almost any water you put into it. Our constipated patient drank water faster than her kidneys could process it, but not faster than her small intestine could absorb it. The end result was blood dilution that could have been life threatening. And by the way, her constipation didn't relent, despite all the water she drank.

There's a special exception: you can add water to fiber as a constipation treatment, as the fiber will hold the water thus causing the stool to retain more moisture. This procedure, however, won't work for SIBO patients because the fiber causes bloating.

There are some new "fad" diets that may help SIBO, such as the popular 18-hour fast, in which you eat only two to three times a week. In our practices, however, we don't recommend eating this way. As previously mentioned, if you eat nothing, your SIBO will improve, but everyone has to eat!

If you have IBS or SIBO, we recommend you eat two or three distinct meals a day, four or five hours apart. This doesn't mean you should be eating less, just less often.

General Nutrition Guidelines

Now that you have a better understanding of how the gastrointestinal tract operates, you know that it's possible to help manage SIBO through your diet. When planning meals, follow the guidelines for foods to choose and foods to avoid in the Appendix at the end of this book. Below are some sample menus to help you plan meals.

BREAKFAST

- One whole egg, plus egg white from a second egg, scrambled. One slice of rye or sourdough bread. You can substitute scrambled eggs for a poached egg on top of a sourdough English muffin with sautéed spinach.
- Berries (handful)
- Tea or coffee with Lactaid milk

or

- Crispy rice cereal with Lactaid milk
- Sliced berries with sprinkling of chopped walnuts
- Tea or coffee with Lactaid milk
- Water

or

- Lactaid cottage cheese with one-half papaya
- One sourdough English muffin
- Sliced stone fruit (optional)
- Tea or coffee with Lactaid milk

LUNCH

- Baked salmon over white rice with tomato, onion, zucchini, and bell pepper sautéed in olive oil
- Pineapple and orange fruit salad
- Water (Crystal Light with aspartame, optional)

or

- Open-faced sandwich: sliced fresh turkey with avocado slices on rye, sourdough, potato, or French bread
- Add a slice of hard cheese, such as aged cheddar (optional)
- Side of a small cucumber and tomato salad with balsamic dressing
- One serving of fruit

or

- Corn tortillas
- One or two slices of oven-roasted turkey
- One sliver of avocado

or

- Leftovers from cooking the night before. (This is a huge help for lunch at work or at home.)

DINNER

- Salmon seasoned with lemon, salt, and pepper
- Frozen corn sautéed with onions and olive oil
- Four or five fresh tomatoes, chopped
- Fresh basil
- Grill salmon until medium rare. Add corn and tomatoes to a sauté pan for five minutes. Add fresh chopped basil. Place grilled salmon on top of corn-tomato mixture on plate.
- White wine

or

- Roast whole chicken with carrots and baby potatoes
- Season a whole chicken with olive oil. Add one teaspoon each of salt, pepper, and paprika (for coloring on outside of chicken). Add a splash of orange juice or white wine (optional).
- Add cut carrots and baby potatoes around the chicken in the same pot
- Cook at 375°F for 1½ hours (check for doneness)
- Serve over white rice (optional)

or

- Chicken with eggplant and salad
- Squeeze juice from one lemon on the outside of a whole chicken cut into parts. Grill chicken parts on medium-hot fire. Spread potato wedges sprinkled with rosemary around the sides of the grill.
- Bake eggplant, sliced length-wise, at 350°F with lemon juice and chopped garlic until tender
- Prepare a small side salad with lettuce. Dress with olive oil, red wine vinegar, and ground black pepper. Add cherry tomatoes and slices of avocado and cucumber (peeled).
- Water

or

- Oven-roasted winter root vegetables
- Peel carrots and parsnips, chop roughly and place in a bowl. Add in roughly chopped yams and potatoes. Toss with olive oil and season with sea salt and pepper. Roast in the oven on a cookie sheet at 400°F for 20 minutes. Sprinkle top with fresh Italian parsley.

Tweaking Low-Fermentation Eating

"I can't eat veggies," said Beth, a 56-year-old lawyer. *"They make me bloated. Every time I go to a salad bar, I'm stumped as to what I can eat."*

Vegetables You don't have to eliminate vegetables from your diet if you have IBS! In the carbohydrate realm of vegetables, it's okay to eat vegetables like eggplant, tomato, and zucchini. We suggest that you eat what we call the "root and fruit" foods, as they don't cause much trouble for IBS or SIBO patients. If you want a salad, instead of using lettuce, try a Greek or Shirazi salad with cucumber, tomato, and a small amount of onion.

Root vegetables, such as potatoes, beets, and carrots, tend to be simpler carbohydrates. Sweet potato has more fiber and is on our optional list. Bell pepper is technically a fruit and is also okay to eat.

You can mix a small amount of onion (as a flavoring ingredient) with ground beef for a burger. Small amounts of garlic also are acceptable. You can also use salt, pepper, and turmeric for seasoning.

Some SIBO patients can tolerate small amounts of garlic. Garlic has many health benefits in addition to digestive benefits, as it's an antioxidant and anti-inflammatory. Individualized attention to each person's diet is important and the reason not to have tunnel vision with your diet for overall health. Some patients with IBS and SIBO eliminate garlic because they think they shouldn't eat it at all because it's banned from the low-FODMAP diet.

Protein Proteins, such as beef, chicken, or fish, are allowed in low-fermentation eating, but if you eat in a restaurant they may be cooked in butter or other banned products, so be cautious and be sure to ask your server how the dish is prepared. We hope that the menu is obvious and that you don't need to ask; for example, a club sandwich is perfectly okay to eat.

We suggest avoiding dairy products because lactose is a difficult sugar to digest. There are many lactose-free options available today. Most SIBO patients can handle lactose-free milk, cheese, or ice cream, but be sure there's no added sucralose in ice cream or gelato.

If you like cheese, go for hard, aged cheese, such as cheddar, Gouda, and Asiago. These cheeses have been fermented for years in some cases and generally have no lactose left. Gruyère cheese is acceptable if it is 100 percent lactose-free and gluten-free. Avoid soft cheeses, such as burrata or cream cheese. Vegan cheese is also usually well tolerated by SIBO patients. Be careful that the alternative cheese is not made with soy, which is a protein to avoid.

Alcohol Can you drink alcohol with low-fermentation eating? Yes, but be aware that mixed drinks may have agave syrup, sucralose, or stevia. If the drink is mixed with soda, make sure there are no artificial sugars in the soda. Bitters are generally well tolerated, so a few drops are fine.

In general, IBS patients tend to tolerate white wine better than red wine, as well as less hoppy and lighter beers—such as lagers or pilsners—rather than stouts or heavy, hoppy ales.

Special Situations

Certain special situations make it imperative to stick to low-fermentation eating as much as possible.

AIR TRAVEL

When you fly long distances, both your brain *and* your gut become jet-lagged. Upsetting your circadian rhythms doesn't just affect brain function, but gut function as well. It takes a while for your bowels to adjust to long-distance travel; you may experience more challenges and bloating. Think about it this way: The cleaning waves of the gut are in part circadian. They occur mostly at night when you sleep. If you've traveled halfway around the world, your day and night are flipped, which can dysregulate the cleaning waves.

Some of our SIBO patients have tried taking melatonin (a hormone that regulates the sleep-wake cycle) to avoid jet lag, but they maintain that their results are mediocre. We recommend that you try to adjust as fast as you can to the time zone you're in. For example, if you know when you land it's going to be dinnertime, plan to eat food on the plane as lunch. Remember, you need to leave four to five hours between meals (Figure 8.1).

Air pressure is also a factor. The pilot will adjust the air pressure once you're up in the air, but the correction isn't 100 percent perfect. That's why your ears pop. Air becomes trapped in the middle ear and as air pressure is lowered, the air in the middle ear expands and you feel pressure. If you yawn or swallow you can balance the pressure via the eustachian tubes in your ear so that the pressure in your ear is the same as inside the plane, at which point the pressure in your ear disappears.

Your small intestine doesn't have that luxury. If you have a lot of gas in your small intestine, when the plane goes up, the gas expands and you may become severely bloated. You can't belch or pass gas. The key is to board the plane with the least amount of gas in your small intestine. Often, IBS patients avoid eating two to four hours before flying, if possible.

If you must eat, do so when the plane is at a stable altitude (when they tell you that you can use large electronic devices), not just after you've boarded. Be sure to take your own food onboard; most airports have good, healthy food available now. On the plane, you're likely to find only low-quality snacks. The ultimate irony of flying is they put you on a plane where the air pressure is lower, and then they offer you a soda or snack boxes of lentil chips with hummus dip. Neither is good for a SIBO patient and will only make your abdomen bulge with gas.

HIGH ALTITUDE

If you have IBS or SIBO and you are at 8000 to 10,000 feet, you'll likely feel bloated with a distended abdomen and you may have SIBO symptoms. The effects of high altitude are similar to flying long distance. Recognize that, at first, you may not feel your best at high altitude, and make good choices. Adherence to low-fermentation eating is even more important.

SHIFT WORK

Shift workers who work the day shift one week and the night shift the following week often have a hard time with their gut rhythms. The more we learn about body clock genes, the more we realize that it's almost impossible for shift workers to follow a diet that keeps cleaning waves intact. Just like long distance travel, your body clock shifts during shift work and it doesn't know when cleaning waves are coming.

Apart from the direct effect of sleep on gut motility, sleep is also very important in regulation of appetite and what we crave to eat. Sleep

Figure 8.1 Meal spacing protocol for diet management of SIBO.

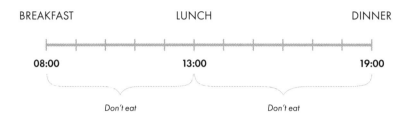

deprivation leads to decreased levels of leptin and an increased level of ghrelin hormones. The net effect is an increased appetite. For reasons that we don't yet understand, sleep deprivation also increases *endocannabinoids*, which increase our craving for fat and sugar, similar to increased appetite with marijuana use ("the munchies"). This change in food consumption behavior has deleterious effects on SIBO and the gut microbiome.

To avoid bloating, shift workers with SIBO need to stick to a plan. When they're awake, they need to engage in low-fermentation eating. When they are off work, they need to find a time to fast for eight hours, even if they're not sleeping.

RELIGIOUS FASTING

For religious fasts, such as the Jewish 25-hour fast of Yom Kippur, we generally recommend that you not overeat or eat too quickly when you break the fast. Hydration is also important. Many people start with a sweet drink or juice. We recommend water instead. The majority of the food served at a break-fast contain carbohydrates, as people believe they need to raise their blood sugar quickly. This is a fallacy, unless you are diabetic. A balanced, high-protein diet is best for breaking a fast.

During the Muslim month of Ramadan, people wake up early before sunrise and eat nothing throughout the day. In the evening after sundown, they have a meal. We recommend good hydration and a high-protein, relatively low-carbohydrate diet. Grilled meat and chicken are good food choices; hummus is not a good idea for someone with IBS.

Stressful Situations

"My IBS would flare up during my final exams," said Robert, a 23-year-old medical student. *"I stayed up late studying, and only got a few hours of sleep. I kept awake by drinking soda and coffee, and I ordered a pizza to be delivered at 3:00 A.M. while I was studying. I was also snacking constantly."*

Common stressful situations, such as an exam, job interview, hospitalization of a loved one, a wedding/engagement party, or parties in general can also affect your gut's balance. When under stress, we frequently change dietary and sleeping habits, which may lead to a change in bowel habits. We may snack more, especially with sweets, sleep less, eat unhealthy foods, and exercise less. For the most part, these changes in your daily routine are the main cause of IBS flare-ups in a stressful situation. Robert, our medical student, would have had an IBS flare-up regardless of the exam because of the acute changes that he made in his daily routine. We suggest you don't change your dietary habits, eat as healthily as you can, avoid snacking, avoid sodas, and drink water to hydrate.

If you know from previous experience that your symptoms may be extremely severe, for example, a bout of diarrhea before a job interview, we recommend you eat an early dinner the night before the interview and then fast for eight to ten hours. You can have water and coffee in the morning before the interview.

If you have severe IBS and are getting married in a month, engage in low-fermentation eating, or you can consider an elemental diet. You'll likely want to lose weight and have a flat belly. The elemental diet will help you achieve both goals while helping control symptoms. This is an extreme option, but it works for stressful events that you know are happening in a few weeks.

At a wedding, or any parties that serve food, appetizers may be offered continually. Avoid food that contains cheese and try not to overeat. Good options include beef sliders or a skewer of shrimp or chicken. For tapas, stick with dishes that are mostly protein. Select crackers with prosciutto, sausage, chicken, or shrimp. If you drink alcohol, clean cocktails—rather than mixed drinks—are good options.

Athletes

Johnny, a star running back who had just graduated from high school, was asked to gain 20 pounds by the college football coach who had recruited him. *"To bulk up, he suggested I drink two liters of milk every day. Coach said I had to gain weight if I wanted to be a starter. He wasn't concerned about me working out and gaining muscle as much as just being heavier,"* said Johnny, who was diagnosed with SIBO at age 17. *"I knew I couldn't drink regular milk or I would get bloated. So I drank lactose-free milk, spread out through the day in three chunks, and gained 15 pounds. Coach was happy and I made the team."*

A number of facets of athletics can make it more complicated to follow low-fermentation eating. We have patients who are body builders, or training for long-distance road races, or who do yoga regularly. They all have different nutritional needs depending on the intensity of their training. If you're a weekend warrior or a more casual exerciser, you don't have to change your diet much. But if you're actively training or competing, or doing high-intensity physical activity regularly, food choice can be a challenge for SIBO patients. You'll require more carbohydrates to fuel activity during training, and you may feel the need to eat more frequently. As we've stated, it's better to eat bigger meals less frequently to avoid bloating and abdominal distention.

If you're an athlete, you may have to eat larger meals three times a day, but you don't want to run a marathon with your stomach packed with food. You have to find a natural balance. Once you stop eating for the day, you *must* stop eating until you have breakfast the next morning. If you're a SIBO patient, we suggest you maximize the amount of continuous time between meals. Don't eat for eight hours overnight. If you wake up at 2:00 A.M. for a bite to eat, bacterial overgrowth may ensue.

Rehydration Drinks

Drinks designed to rehydrate are a particular challenge for SIBO/IBS patients. These drinks usually contain fructose or high-fructose corn syrup in combination with glucose to give you more energy; however, at the same time they tend to cause bloating, gas, and abdominal distention. Even people without SIBO who drink two Gatorades at once may have some bloating. Some manufacturers put inulin (fiber) into energy drinks without informing consumers, and as previously discussed, this fiber can also cause bloating, gas, and abdominal distention. Be cautious about what is in your energy drink: read the label. If you're running a 10K race or a marathon, choose your hydration and energy sources carefully. You're more likely to underperform during the race if you feel bloated because of SIBO.

JUICING

Fad diets, like juicing, are popular with athletes, but juicing may not be a good thing. Juices often contain too much carbohydrate: fructose, in particular. Green juices may be high in green, leafy fiber, which may also precipitate bloating and abdominal distention. We're not implying that juicing is unhealthy, but it may not be practical for SIBO patients because of their tendency to bloat.

AVOIDING BLOATING AND DISTENTION

Bloating and abdominal distention can be a tremendous hindrance to endurance. If you're bloated because of something you drank or ate on race day, your oxygen transfer may be compromised due to pressure below the diaphragm. The distention makes breathing a little more labored and that can impact your ability to compete. That's another reason to minimize bloating.

Runners usually fast on race day to minimize bloating. This is a double-edged sword for those of you with SIBO. You don't want to be bloated on race day as your oxygen exchange will be less efficient. But if you fast you may not have enough carbohydrates available to provide quick energy. If you follow the rules of low-fermentation eating, your body will have enough stored carbohydrates, even for a long event. That's your best bet.

You may also take a tip from professional hockey players. If you're a hockey fan, you may have seen professional players between shifts squirt liquid from a bottle into their mouths and then spit it out without swallowing. The glucose in the drink is absorbed under the tongue and the carbohydrates in the drink provide an extra boost of energy. This procedure may be helpful for SIBO patients because you don't actually drink and absorb the sugars during competition. If you swish and spit without drinking, you get the carbohydrates you need, but you don't feed the bacteria in the gut. Use only a pure glucose drink, which may be difficult to find.

Some athletes drink protein shakes to bulk up, but most commercial protein powders contain sucralose or other unacceptable artificial sweeteners. Manufacturers use these non-absorbable sweeteners to make the drink more palatable, but you may feel bloated all day. Look for a protein shake with glucose or dextrose, not fructose, sucralose, or sorbitol, and nothing with prebiotics like inulin. We recommend whey protein isolate, which is derived from milk. If it's pure whey protein, it shouldn't have much lactose. For vegan athletes, we recommend pea protein.

Vegans

Vegan patients with SIBO present a challenging situation. Their essential energy sources are carbohydrates and soy protein, both of which are challenging foods for SIBO patients. A lot of vegans rely on lentils and beans as protein sources, which are not good food sources for SIBO patients. In general, vegans have a hard time following any IBS diet.

OPTIONS

However, vegans do have options. Low-fermentation eating allows vegetable protein, such as pea protein, which is now readily available and is more palatable than other pure vegetable-based proteins. Nuts and nut butters that do not contain sweeteners are also a good source of protein for vegans. Nut butters are often sweetened, so look at the label for the type of sugar and avoid any products with fructose or sucralose. Low-fermentation eating allows some vegetables and fruits. (See the Appendix.)

Vegans often feel hungry because it takes the stomach a long time to crush, grind, and break-down vegetable-derived protein and fat. They don't get a sense of feeling full and may feel hungry two to three hours after eating. This hunger can lead to a habit of grazing throughout the day, which sets them up for potential bacterial overgrowth. Vegans with SIBO should try to space their meals as much as possible to allow for cleaning waves.

Vegetarians

It's a little easier for vegetarians with SIBO. Depending on the type of vegetarianism you practice, you can have milk and eggs or fish and seafood. For food sources, the same principles apply as to vegans, except that the protein sources are more plentiful. Low-fermentation eating allows lactose-free dairy, and you can even bake with lactose-free milk. Eggs or egg whites are another tremendous source of protein and energy. To limit the amount of fat in your diet, use egg whites instead of whole eggs. Whey protein is another good choice.

The best protein sources for vegetarians with SIBO include lactose-free cottage cheese, nuts, peanut butter, almonds, and green peas. Hemp, chia seeds, and quinoa, in small quantities, may be acceptable. Just as with vegans, lentils and beans are not acceptable for SIBO patients.

Our vegan and vegetarian patients are very creative and they challenge us to learn about new sources of protein. They'll go to a natural food store and find unique foods that the average person doesn't know about, such as spelt. Spelt is an ancient grain that's similar to wheat and is an excellent source protein, dietary fiber, several B vitamins, and numerous minerals. You can eat spelt in small quantities with low-fermentation eating, but spelt is a fiber, so you can't eat too much of it. We work with our patients to individually customize and monitor their diets to ascertain how much spelt they can tolerate.

Diabetics

For diabetes patients who have IBS/SIBO, our general recommendation is to avoid fermentable foods, however, a heart-healthy diet usually relies on lots of fiber and green vegetables to protect your heart against potential damage from diabetes. This may lead to bloating if you eat excessive amounts of vegetables and fruits.

Many dietitians are familiar with diets for diabetes, high blood pressure, and heart conditions, but not as familiar with diets for gastrointestinal disorders. Search for a dietitian who is familiar with IBS-related diets and diabetes, and share with them the details of low-fermentation eating. Let your primary care physician know about your food choices as well.

Diabetics on a low-sugar diet are told to avoid high-fructose containing foods, which aligns with low-fermentation eating. We offer many healthy options in low-fermentation eating that are good for diabetics, including green vegetables, such as such as kale, spinach, and arugula, as well as raspberries, blueberries, and blackberries. Avoid mulberries due to their high-fructose content. If you have SIBO, you should minimize some vegetables usually recommended in a diabetic diet, including cabbage, romaine lettuce, cauliflower, and legumes. You can substitute other heathy options. See the Low-Fermentation Eating Guide Appendix at the back of this book.

If you become hypoglycemic and need sugar quickly, use a glucose drink or glucose tablets, which are absorbed in the mouth and don't reach the small intestine. This will raise your blood sugar, you won't feel bloated, and you won't activate an eating phase in the gastrointestinal tract.

The Low-Fermentation Eating Way of Life

If you follow the straightforward rules of low-fermentation eating—avoid non-digestible sugars and space your meals—you'll find it's an easy plan to stick to. If you accidentally eat something outside the plan, don't panic. You won't provoke bacterial overgrowth with one or two deviations, although you may be bloated for 24 hours. If, however, you are off the plan consistently, you will trigger significant bacterial overgrowth.

The point of low-fermentation eating is not to drive you insane—just relax and live a normal life. We don't want you to be stressed about what you can or can't eat.

We've been prescribing low-fermentation eating for almost 20 years. This plan is effective at maintaining good nutrition while providing relief from SIBO symptoms, but we want to emphasize that diet alone won't cure SIBO. Even if you strictly follow low-fermentation eating, diet alone is not going to get rid of bacterial overgrowth.

SIBO management takes multiple forms. By far, the most complex and challenging is diet. It can be confusing for both patients and doctors. We all have to to deal with diet on a daily basis, for one reason or another. Low-fermentation eating alone won't fix your SIBO, but it will give you clarification and guidelines on how to handle SIBO.

Depending on your underlying pathophysiology, the severity of your symptoms, and how compliant you are with the plan, improvement ranges dramatically, from 10 percent to 70 percent. Eighty to ninety percent of our patients see some improvement with low-fermentation eating. Patients who have minimal or no improvement may have other accompanying problems to consider.

The next chapter describes what you can do if you're not feeling better after managing your SIBO and changing your diet.

CHAPTER 9

I'm Not All Better. Now What Do I Do?

More than a decade ago, the patients referred to us were less exposed to microbiome-based therapies and therefore easier to treat. Nowadays things have changed for the better. Many doctors are now using therapies like the antibiotic rifaximin earlier in their patient care. However, the type of patients we now see are more complicated, as they've failed the first-line therapies. All of our patients have seen other doctors, including gastroenterologists, who have not been able to resolve their IBS or SIBO problems. These tougher-to-treat cases can at first seem bleak. There are, however, other modalities to help them feel better.

When we get to this point, depending on your symptoms, we use a more in-depth history and physical examination to pick up clues that you may have something besides IBS or SIBO, or a concomitant factor that adds to your scenario. We'll generally ask, "What bothers you most?" Some of our patients still have diarrhea even with SIBO treatment. Others experience no diarrhea, but still feel bloated, or they have diarrhea, but no bloating. For those with constipation, their abdominal distention may be improved, but they continue to have a sensation of incomplete evacuation.

We look for a specific cause for a specific symptom in patients who are not responding to standard SIBO management. There are some drugs that can target these symptoms and improve them. This chapter covers the additional therapies we use for patients who don't respond to our standard IBS/SIBO treatment protocol. The following therapies are not miracles, but they may help if you're still in need of relief. We'll also discuss diseases other than IBS and SIBO that may cause or contribute to your symptoms.

Peppermint

Peppermint has been known to help IBS symptoms for some time, and we've seen it work for our own IBS patients.

Peppermint appears to work in multiple ways. It is a calcium channel blocker. Calcium channels are fundamental to vascular muscle (muscle in the walls of blood vessels). Calcium channel blockers are often prescribed for people with heart disease, as they relax affected blood vessels, thus reducing blood pressure.

Peppermint works as a topical agent in the gastrointestinal tract. It blocks calcium channels in the smooth muscle from the esophagus all the way to the rectum (if it gets that far), and relaxes muscles as it travels. If you take even a small amount of peppermint by mouth, the active ingredient (L-menthol) allows the spice sensors in your mouth to feel the coolness. By relaxing the gut muscles, it can relieve cramping.

Peppermint tea may help your IBS symptoms, but it's not clear whether it can affect the small intestine because most of the peppermint is quickly absorbed. If you respond to peppermint tea, but continue to have symptoms, you may respond better to a peppermint oil formulation. There are a number of enteric coated formulations of peppermint oil that allow it to be released in the small intestine. We've seen it help with IBS symptoms of bloating, diarrhea, and abdominal cramps. You have to take it multiple times a day, but it may take the edge off your symptoms.

Peppermint oil is also one of the best treatments for esophageal spasm. If you experience an esophageal spasm, mix four drops of peppermint oil with water and drink it to relax your esophagus.

Peppermint can also affect serotonin receptors, which occur throughout the body but are particularly plentiful in the brain and the gut. The most important receptors in the gut are 5-HT3 and 5-HT4. When activated, these serotonin receptors make the bowels move faster. When they're blocked, the gut slows down. Peppermint is a weak 5-HT3 antagonist and can help with IBS diarrhea. A peppermint oil formulation has been shown to improve IBS diarrhea in a robust, randomized controlled trial, but more rigorous studies are needed to determine its effectiveness and safety.

Finally, in some small studies, peppermint has been shown to have antibacterial properties, and may reduce bacteria in SIBO.

Serotonin Blockers

The 5-HT3 receptor antagonists, also called serotonin receptor antagonists or serotonin blockers, are in a class of medicines that are used for the prevention and treatment of nausea and vomiting caused by chemotherapy, radiation therapy, or post-surgery. Serotonin blockers were, in fact, initially developed to treat the nausea and vomiting associated with chemotherapy, and when used during cancer treatment, most patients' nausea improved dramatically.

Some common 5-HT3 receptor antagonists include dolasetron, granisetron, and ondansetron. Despite variations in their chemical structures and absorption rates, they all work in the same way and are well tolerated by most patients. The oral formulations of these drugs are just as effective as the intravenous forms at preventing nausea and vomiting.

An oral version of these drugs can also be used for gastrointestinal problems. The drugs help some patients with IBS diarrhea because they slow down the gut. If you have IBS diarrhea, you'll need to take one of the above serotonin blockers one to three times a day.

A potent 5-HT3 antagonist, alosetron, was one of the first drugs approved for IBS diarrhea in 2000. When it was introduced, some patients with severe diarrhea-prominent IBS found it to be too strong. While uncommon, some patients (less than one percent) also developed ischemic colitis (reduced blood flow to the colon that causes tissue to begin to die), and for this reason it was temporarily taken off the market. Due to a significant unmet need and with the addition of a safety management program, it was reintroduced in 2002 with a more restricted indication and a requirement that doctors and patients follow a prescribing program. It is now only allowed for women with severe diarrhea IBS who have failed conventional therapy. We only use alosetron if you've tried, and failed, multiple medications. If you're prescribed alosetron, make sure you're aware of the side effects.

We rarely prescribe alosetron because there are other effective sero-tonin blockers that don't carry the risk of severe side effects. We prefer to prescribe ondansetron over alosetron.

Antihistamines

Occasionally, bowel sensitivity is due to the hyperactivity of mast cells and other allergy-related cells. Mast cells mediate inflammatory responses, such as hypersensitivity and allergic reactions. These cells cause allergic symptoms by releasing products called "mediators" that are either stored inside them or manufactured by them. Mast cells produce more than 200 mediators, histamine being one of the most common. Interestingly, a study from UZ Leuven led by Dr. Guy Boeckxstaens suggests that infectious gastroenteritis can lead to a local allergic reaction, leading to abdominal pain, suggesting that microbes in the gut can also change our tolerance to food and lead to specific food allergies.

Antihistamines are designed to counteract the effects of histamine. Second-generation antihistamines, such as Zyrtec, Claritin, and Allegra, don't cause the drowsiness side-effect of the first-generation antihistamines, and may help if IBS symptoms are related to mast cells. In those cases, patients appear to harbor a large amount of histamine, which may be a cause of heightened abdominal pain. In some patients, microbiome-activating cells produce mediators, including histamine. If you can't decrease your symptoms by modifying your microbiome, adding antihistamines to your treatment may help. These treatments, however, require care and monitoring by a specialist in mast cell activation syndrome. We have published a detailed peer-reviewed guide for gastroenterologists who are interested in patients with mast cell activation syndrome.

We know of one controlled study that showed that the mast cell stabilizer ketotifen, rather than the placebo in the study, increased the threshold for discomfort in IBS patients with abdominal pain, reduced IBS symptoms, and improved health-related quality of life. Other mast cell stabilizers, such as cromolyn, as well as a combination of multiple drugs, may also be considered in this situation.

GCC Agonists

Guanylate Cyclase C (GCC) agonists are approved treatments for constipation. The FDA has approved two drugs: linaclotide and plecanatide. In the 1970s, scientists wondered why people developed diarrhea from *E. coli* even though those bacteria don't cause direct injury to the bowel lining. They found that *E. coli* bacteria produce a toxin that leads to profuse diarrhea. This led to the discovery of GCC receptors in the gut. When activated, these receptors push sodium, bicarbonate and chloride, from the cells lining the gut. This pushes water from the body into the gut, thus causing diarrhea.

When we run out of options for patients with IBS constipation, we give them a GCC agonist to increase fluid in the lumen of the gut, essentially giving them diarrhea, and their constipation generally improves. Please note that this therapy doesn't address the underlying cause of constipation. It's also difficult to balance the dose. If you give too much drug, the patient may have too much diarrhea, whereas if you give too little, it doesn't clear the constipation.

Other Drug Treatments

A handful of other drug treatments may also work in certain situations, especially if nothing else stems the tide of IBS symptoms.

Lubiprostone. This medication is used in the management of chronic constipation. A derivative of prostaglandin E1, it activates chloride channels in epithelial cells lining the gut. Lubiprostone brings water into the gut, similar to GCC agonists, and is used in IBS constipation. It's not quite as effective as GCC agonists.

5-HT4 serotonin agonists (activators). If taken during a fasting state, these drugs activate the cleaning waves and colon movements to move food through the gut to help control constipation. One 5-HT4 serotonin agonist, cisapride, proved very effective; however, as with any serotonin activator, it affected 5-HT receptors in the heart. This led to heart arrhythmias and was pulled from the market. Another 5-HT4 drug, tegaserod, was less concerning. In a review of cumulative data, heart attacks and strokes were rare, but based on uncertainty the drug was pulled pending further study. After extended safety trials, tegaserod was reapproved in mid-2019 for women under age 65, but it came with a box warning that it may cause cardiovascular events, dehydration, ischemic colitis, and a small, but significant, signal of suicidal ideation. If you've tried everything and you are still suffering with constipation, tegaserod may be an option, but you'll need to be monitored by your doctor.

Prucalopride. A safer drug for constipation is prucalopride, which has the highest affinity for 5HT-4 receptors, and has been approved to treat constipation in the US, Europe, Canada, and Australia. Rigorous drug testing ruled out increased cardiac effects, but it does have a box warning for suicidal ideation. If you take prucalopride and you feel depressed or suicidal, stop taking the drug immediately and see your doctor. We often use this drug as nighttime dosing for SIBO as recurrence prevention. Daytime dosing works better for chronic constipation. Although prucalopride is FDA-approved, it remains difficult to get until insurance coverage improves.

Mu-receptor agonists. Morphine is the prototypical mu-opioid receptor agonist. Mu-receptors are a class of opioid receptors that are also referred to as mu-opioid peptide receptors. When these receptors are activated, the gut slows down and abdominal pain improves. Mu-receptor agonists, such as eluxadoline, are approved for IBS with diarrhea. In addition, eluxadoline carries a box warning because it can lead to pancreatitis, a potentially severe inflammation of the pancreas. This drug can be very effective if used in the correct patient, but cannot be used if the patient has gallstones, history of gallbladder removal, pancreatitis, or excessive alcohol ingestion.

Over-the-counter mu-receptor agonists. Imodium is a shorter-acting and weaker version of eluxadoline. We generally don't recommend SIBO patients take Imodium because it slows down the gut. If you're going to an important meeting and you have diarrhea, you may take one or two Imodium tablets to allow you to hold on through the meeting. Lomotil is a slightly longer-acting mu-receptor agonist, but requires a prescription.

Opium tincture. Also known as laudanum, this liquid is made of air-dried poppy and it contains morphine and codeine as well. It's one of the oldest medications in medicine. It's generally prescribed as an antidiarrheal agent to slow transit of the intestines by increasing intestinal smooth muscle tone and inhibiting motility. Water is absorbed from fecal contents, decreasing diarrhea. Since this is a true opiate, the potential for abuse and addiction is high.

Anticholinergics. Anticholinergics, such as dicyclomine, are used for immediate pain relief of stomach cramps from IBS. Another anticholinergic, hyoscyamine, fights spasms in the gut and can treat muscle cramps in the bowels as well as the symptoms of IBS, colitis, and other digestive problems. These drugs help reduce symptoms by slowing the natural movements of the gut and by relaxing the muscles in the stomach and intestines. Anticholinergics control symptoms, but they don't address what causes your IBS.

L-glutamine. This abundant amino acid, produced by the body and also found in food, may heal the lining of the bowel and help with IBS symptoms. A recent medium-sized randomized controlled trial found 5000 mg doses (about 2 teaspoons) of L-glutamine three times daily improved IBS symptoms and intestinal permeability, the so-called leaky gut. Larger trials are needed to confirm this data. L-glutamine is a safe supplement and an option for IBS treatment and potentially for leaky gut. Make sure you take a pure L-glutamine supplement with no other compounds.

Fiber Supplements

It's almost an urban myth that if you eat more fiber, your bowel habits will be perfect. The largest fiber study ever done, with more than 10,000 patients, found no association between a low intake of fiber and constipation. Fiber does have other health benefits, and currently the FDA has approved two fiber supplements with lipid-lowering properties—psyllium and beta glucan.

Psyllium. From a gastrointestinal standpoint, fiber can relieve constipation for some people; however, some studies show that eating more fiber makes constipation worse. Psyllium is a gel-forming soluble fiber derived from the husks of the psyllium seed. When it reaches the gut, it becomes a gel and traps water, and it doesn't allow bile acid to reabsorb. The majority of bile acid, which is produced by the liver, is reabsorbed at the end of the small intestine and then recycled by the body so that the liver doesn't have to work as hard to produce more bile acid. With less bile acid, the liver has to use cholesterol to produce more bile acid, which reduces your body's cholesterol level by a small amount. From an IBS standpoint, increased bile acid in the colon can cause symptoms. Bloating is a common complaint of our IBS patients who take psyllium, which is found in Metamucil. The good news is that, as far as we know, psyllium is not fermentable and bacteria can't break it down. We have patients who say they become distended and pass excessive gas when they take psyllium. It's plausible that there may be a bacterium that breaks down psyllium.

Psyllium is usually recommended to adjust your stool consistency more in the middle; that is, not on the diarrhea or the constipation side. If you have bacterial overgrowth, fiber supplements may not help and they may even cause problems. They have no properties to help with your pain, urgency, or abdominal distention; they can only improve the consistency of your stool. Stool consistency is generally not the main complaint of SIBO patients. Insoluble fibers, such as bran and rye, don't absorb water. Bran may or may not decrease cholesterol levels, but it definitely makes almost everyone feel bloated and distended if eaten in large quantities. Bran is not a good idea for SIBO patients. Other fiber types are soluble but fermentable, such as inulin or fructo-oligosaccharides. As we've described, after ingestion they are fermented in your gut. Inulin is a classic fructan, and can cause significant bloating and distention in IBS/SIBO patients.

Calcium polycarbophil. Another fiber option is the synthetic fiber calcium polycarbophil, which is not fermented by bacteria. It can cause bloating, but we occasionally use it to improve the stool form. We don't expect patients' abdominal pain or distention to go away, but their stool may look better.

Other Laxatives

Other medications used to treat occasional constipation are known as osmotic-type laxatives, including Miralax and multiple generic brands available over the counter. These laxatives work by holding water in the stool, which softens the stool and increases the number of bowel movements. They are composed of polyethylene glycol (PEG) 3350, which sounds like antifreeze, but it's actually a synthetic molecule not associated with antifreeze. Once consumed, the molecules pull water into the gastrointestinal tract to help with the consistency of your stools if you're constipated. It also suctions water from the small intestine, which keeps the colon moist.

Polyethylene glycol 3350 is not absorbed by humans or by bacteria; it maintains its integrity until it leaves the body by defecation. Water stays with it, making the stool looser. Because it won't feed bacteria, we occasionally use it to get things moving for constipated SIBO patients. Polyethylene glycol has no side effects or drug interactions; it simply causes your stool to become slightly looser, which leads to less straining during defecation, although you may have to clean up more afterward due to the loose consistency of stool. Polyethylene glycol 3350 is also the main ingredient in the drinks used to clean your bowels before a colonoscopy. We know this molecule is safe because it's been used in high doses before colonoscopy, and it doesn't dehydrate or affect the kidneys.

STOOL SOFTENERS

Sometimes we recommend stool softeners to our patients. Their primary ingredient, sodium docusate, makes the surface of the stool more slippery. It has no real role in the management of SIBO, but you can take it to alleviate straining during bowel movements. These stool softeners are often used after surgery, particularly if you've been given pain-killers and narcotics, both of which suck water out of the stool, leaving it hard and dry. Stool softeners generally don't work very well except in mild cases. The body eventually does the work and allows the stool to slip out.

HERBAL REMEDIES

Some of our patients prefer to use herbal remedies for constipation. One commonly used herbal laxative is derived from *senna* leaves in the form of tea, tablets, or suppositories. This laxative stimulates the bowels to push forward, but its action is erratic, and it may cause cramping. If you use it on a regular basis, your bowels will become dependent on it. If the severity of your constipation was 5 on a scale of 1 to 10 and you use senna regularly for one year, you may end up with a constipation level of 8 out of 10. This phenomenon, called rebound constipation, may make your symptoms harder to control. Unfortunately, the rebound constipation associated with this particular herbal laxative may be permanent.

Cascara sagrada has laxative effects similar to senna. In 2002 the FDA banned cascara sagrada as an over-the-counter laxative due to safety concerns, but be aware that it is still added to some supplements. Also note that cascara sagrada is different from cascara that comes from the coffee plant. We do not recommend taking cascara sagrada.

Triphala is an herbal concoction that has been used as a traditional Ayurvedic medicine and healing remedy for more than 1000 years. It consists of three medicinal plants native to India that help the bowels move, but we don't know whether or not triphala activates housekeeping waves. It's milder than the other herbal laxatives, with no known long-term side effects, but there have been no human studies of triphala's effects.

Why We Don't Routinely Use Antidepressants for IBS

Use of antidepressants and antipsychotics for IBS has been advocated by some health-care providers for almost half a century. Despite this, there is no antidepressant or drug with antidepressant/antipsychotic property approved for treatment of IBS by the FDA or European or Asian drug agencies.

The idea of using antidepressant medications for IBS is challenging. For one, it indirectly implies that patients with IBS have a psychological origin to their disease. In fact, there is no level one data from prospective trials to show a cause-and-effect relationship between psychological events and IBS.

Another problem with the use of antidepressants in IBS is the poor data quality. While there have been randomized controlled studies using these drugs, the majority have failed to demonstrate benefit. When this happens in the drug industry, researchers tend to conduct what is called a meta-analysis. This occurs when all the studies of particular type are pooled. This is like taking 10 studies and pooling the data to reveal what the data would have looked like if there were one big study. There are many problems with this approach. Small studies that are negative are less often published, so those aren't included. Also, each study uses different methods. But the largest problem for antidepressants studies is that the trials use different drugs (some use amitriptyline, some desipramine, and so on). It's a little like pooling fruit and including apples and oranges together. Despite these limitations, in the end these meta-analyses show that there may be some benefit to using these drugs to treat IBS.

Another consideration with antidepressants is the way they work. When used for gut problems, they're generally not working as antidepressants. For example, tricyclic antidepressants have a constipating side effect, so the reason people with IBS feel better is because the side effect of another drug is making their diarrhea better.

It's also important to consider safety when prescribing this category of medication. Among IBS drugs, a recent harm study conducted by our group pooled the harmful side effects of all drugs to treat IBS. Antidepressants were among the worst. Side effects of tricyclic antidepressants include dry mouth, constipation (enough to stop the drug), heart rhythm problems, and impotence, among others. These side effects are not seen with other therapies.

One final note of caution. These medications can have even more side effects and unpredictable events when combined. Some clinicians add one to another or even use three of these drugs together. There's no scientific study using pooled drugs in a randomized study, so this practice is discouraged.

If You Don't Fit the Mold

If you still have IBS symptoms even after attempting these alternative treatments, you may have an overlapping disorder that causes your symptoms. If you're in this category, you may need further testing for other possible disorders. Diagnostic tests include colonoscopy, scans, or x-rays, particularly for younger people.

This section describes diseases that can mimic IBS and SIBO. We mention them, but we don't discuss them in detail. If you have any of these diseases, please seek medical assistance.

CELIAC DISEASE

Celiac disease is a disease of the immune system, but it's not necessarily an autoimmune disease. The most common signs and symptoms of celiac disease include diarrhea, bloating, excess gas, fatigue, weight loss, and iron-deficiency anemia.

If you have celiac disease, your body reacts to gluten, a protein found in wheat. This reaction results in a cascade of physiologic events that diminish the lining of the intestines, causing inflammation. The long, hair-like villi that line the small intestine become inflamed and blunted, even flattened, and as a result food absorption suffers. Some patients develop osteoporosis from poor absorption of nutrients, especially Vitamin D. In severe cases, celiac disease can lead to bowel cancer if left untreated.

The diagnosis of celiac disease requires a blood test. The most accurate marker in the blood is an increase in the antibody to tissue transglutaminase. If this test is positive, the gold standard to diagnose celiac disease is a biopsy of the small intestine through endoscopy. An early diagnosis is decisive for a better prognosis.

Treatment for celiac disease includes complete avoidance of gluten. Many books are available with information about which foods do and don't contain gluten. If you have celiac disease, you'll need medical help to manage it. Some patients develop refractory celiac disease that can lead to a long list of extra-intestinal manifestations that are too numerous to detail in this book.

INFLAMMATORY BOWEL DISEASE

Inflammatory bowel disease (IBD) pertains to two chronic, recurrent diseases of the gastrointestinal tract—ulcerative colitis and Crohn's disease. Both diseases are characterized by chronic inflammation of the gastrointestinal tract. An abnormal microbiome, genetic predisposition, or environmental factors may contribute to the immune dysregulation.

Ulcerative colitis involves a part of the colon or the whole colon, and causes ulcerations of variable severity. It also generally involves the lining of the bowel. Typical symptoms include diarrhea and bloody bowel movements. If you have ulcerative colitis, you have an increased risk of cancer, and you'll need treatment to prevent progression, as well as continual surveillance to ensure the inflammation remains under control.

Crohn's disease dives deeper into tissue. Its inflammation can occur anywhere in the gastrointestinal tract, including the small intestine, colon, and perianal area. Strictures (narrowing) of the bowel are a common complication, as Crohn's disease involves the whole wall of the bowel. It can also cause fistulas, which connect two parts of the bowel to each other, or the bowel to the vagina, bladder, or skin. The symptoms of Crohn's disease are abdominal pain or bloating, diarrhea, or bloody diarrhea. Other symptoms, uncommon in IBS, may include fever, weight loss, and night sweats.

To diagnose IBD, colonoscopy is the mainstay. Your doctor will look at the lining of the bowel for ulcerations and take a biopsy to check for evidence of chronic inflammation. The treatment for IBD includes immunosuppressive, anti-inflammatory drugs.

If you have a family history of IBD, you have up to 10 times the risk of IBD than the general population. As stated earlier in this book, IBD by itself can affect gut motility and complicate bacterial overgrowth. Even though IBD is common, IBS is much more common, so if you have IBD, you may also have IBS. If we treat IBD and heal the ulcers, but your gastrointestinal symptoms remain, you may have IBS on top of IBD. Up to 30 percent of our IBD patients also have IBS. A classic example is a patient with IBS/IBD overlap who's been treated with immunosuppressive drugs that successfully reduced the inflammation and therefore has no bloody bowel movements, anemia, or other common symptoms of inflammation, yet their abdominal pain and bloating remain. We have shown that more than 50 percent of such patients have SIBO.

MICROSCOPIC COLITIS

Microscopic colitis is an inflammation of the colon that causes persistent watery diarrhea. The name derives from the need to examine colon tissue under a microscope, as the tissue appears normal during colonoscopy. The typical microscopic colitis patient is a woman over age 60 with watery diarrhea who has 5 to 15 bowel movements a day.

There are three subtypes of microscopic colitis:

Lymphocytic colitis, in which white blood cells (lymphocytes) increase in colon tissue.

Collagenous colitis, in which a thick layer of protein (collagen) develops in colon tissue.

Incomplete microscopic colitis, in which there are mixed features of collagenous and lymphocytic colitis.

The inflammation of the colon found in microscopic colitis may be due to medications that irritate the lining of the colon, such as proton pump inhibitors and non-steroidal anti-inflammatory agents; bacteria and viruses that produce toxins that irritate the lining of the colon and trigger inflammation; and poor absorption of bile acid.

Treatment modalities for microscopic colitis include corticosteroids, bismuth, and anti-inflammatory medications.

PANCREATIC INSUFFICIENCY

Pancreatic insufficiency occurs when the pancreas doesn't produce enough digestive enzymes to break down food in the intestine. Many diseases, including chronic inflammation of the pancreas, autoimmune diseases, genetic disorders, and long-term alcohol use, can cause the pancreas to become less efficient and to shrink in size. That said, pancreatic insufficiency is very uncommon.

When the pancreas doesn't produce enough enzymes to service the small intestine, food is not digested well. When the undigested food reaches the colon, it is fermented, causing abdominal distention, bloating, and diarrhea due to bacterial overgrowth and SIBO. A lack of the fat enzyme lipase can also cause diarrhea and greasy, oily stool. The chief complaint is significant abdominal pain.

Chronic pancreatitis is diagnosed through imaging scans to assess whether the pancreas is healthy. A low level of the enzyme elastase in the stool may also suggest that the pancreas isn't producing enough digestive enzymes. This test may lead to false-positive results if your stool is watery.

Pancreatic enzyme replacement therapy replaces the pancreatic enzyme with medical-grade supplements.

BILE ACID MALABSORPTION

Bile acids produced by the liver travel through the small intestine and help with the absorption of fat until they are reabsorbed at the end of the small intestine. If bile gets into the colon, it can cause diarrhea, which happens often in Crohn's disease because the end of the small intestine is inflamed or has been surgically resected.

SIBO is another common cause of bile acid malabsorption. The microbiome of the small intestine can affect the binding of bile acids and their reabsorption, and lead to bile acids in the colon and, as a result, diarrhea. So treatment of SIBO can also treat bile acid malabsorption. We may someday be able to modify the small intestine microbiome so that it allows the reabsorption of bile acids.

Treatment of bile acid malabsorption involves use of bile acid sequestrants, such as cholestyramine, colestipol, and colesevelam, which are medications used to lower low-density lipoprotein cholesterol. These medications bind bile acids in the intestine and increase the excretion of bile acids in the stool. However, bile acid sequestrants can bind to and decrease the absorption of other drugs, such as warfarin, thyroid hormones, digoxin, thiazide diuretics, and many others. You need to take other medications one hour before or four to six hours after taking a bile acid sequestrant to avoid interactions.

Of note, there have been no controlled trials for treating bile acid diarrhea in patients, so using this treatment for IBS, for example, is based on poorly controlled trials.

PELVIC FLOOR DYSFUNCTION

Pelvic floor dysfunction is the inability to correctly tighten and relax the pelvic floor muscles to have a bowel movement. Symptoms include constipation, urine or stool leakage, and a frequent need to urinate.

A number of abnormalities can lead to pelvic floor dysfunction. *Hirschsprung's disease* is a congenital nerve disorder of the colon. It's characterized by the absence of particular nerve cells in the bowel. The absence of these nerve cells causes the muscles in the bowels to lose their ability to move stool through the rectum. This condition is usually found in infants.

A more common abnormality is *dyssynergic defecation*, characterized by a difficulty in passing stool due to problems with discoordination of the muscles of the pelvic floor and abdomen. It's as if you're trying to move your bowels and hold them in at the same time. Dyssynergic defecation in some cases can be associated with a previous history of sexual trauma and abuse, and a psychological overlay can precipitate this type of behavior. While the great majority of cases of dyssynergic defection are not associated with history of abuse, your doctor may question you about this possibility. It's important to treat the whole person in these instances. The tragedy of abuse can have lasting effects that necessitate professional care that is beyond the scope of this book.

A mechanical problem with the rectum, such as a kink or prolapse (when the rectum drops down toward or outside your anus), can also be an obstacle to getting stool out, and can lead to constipation. This telescoping of the rectum can cause a rectal ulcer that causes irritability and hypersensitivity. Rectal hypersensitivity occurs if your rectum senses smaller pieces of stool, and you feel the need to go, but there's not much there. The most common cause of pelvic floor injury occurs after delivering a baby. If the injury is significant, it usually causes incontinence, and is not typically associated with constipation or diarrhea. If you have both IBS with diarrhea and a weak anal sphincter or loose pelvis from a pelvic floor dysfunction due to an obstetric injury, you'll likely have diarrhea with gas and stool incontinence.

The treatment for this long list of pelvic floor issues is beyond the scope of this book, but it's important to know that the issues described above can impact your IBS. The pelvic area is very complicated. Testing and imaging can help diagnose a pelvic floor dysfunction, and treatment varies, depending on the cause.

MITOCHONDRIAL DISORDERS

Mitochondrial disorders include a rare group of genetic disorders in which the cells in the body don't produce enough energy, and as a result, the muscles of the gut don't function well. This leads to profound abdominal distention or pain and very bad constipation and bloating. After ruling out a mechanical obstruction or blockage through testing, there may be a functional reason for the distention, what's known as a pseudo-obstruction (not a real obstruction, it's due to a paralyzed muscle). The diagnosis of mitochondrial myopathy is complicated. A muscle biopsy, genetic testing and electromyography can evaluate the electrical activity of muscles. A family history may provide a hint of the disorder. The workup is complicated and this disorder is quite rare. While several supplements are commonly used to treat it, as of now there is no definite treatment for mitochondrial disorders.

SMALL INTESTINAL FUNGAL OVERGROWTH

Fungi and yeast are an important component of the gut microbiome and are also referred to as a mycobiome. The composition, distribution, and diversity of fungal communities in the gut are not well established. We've launched the largest trial to date to define mycobiome in various diseases. The most common fungus in your gut is called *Candida albicans*. Similar to SIBO, fungal elements can overgrow in the small intestine and cause symptoms. The only way to diagnose small intestinal fungal overgrowth (SIFO) is to perform an endoscopic aspiration of the small intestine and culture it for fungal elements. Current stool, saliva, or blood tests are not accurate in diagnosing SIFO. SIFO can be treated with antifungal medications, such as nystatin.

Other Disorders with IBS-Like Symptoms

We've mentioned the following disorders that often appear to mimic IBS symptoms earlier in the book, and we revisit them here.

Mast cell activation syndrome can cause heart, lung, and skin-related symptoms. The gastrointestinal tract symptoms, which may be related to bacterial overgrowth, include diarrhea, nausea with vomiting, and crampy abdominal pain. Patients commonly report multiple allergies.

Ehlers-Danlos syndrome (EDS) is a genetic disorder that weakens the connective tissues of your body. Of the several types of EDS, the type that's commonly associated with gastrointestinal symptoms is called *hypermobile EDS or type 3 EDS*. EDS patients commonly have hyperflexible joints and a history of joint pain and dislocations. These patients may also have bloating, distention, delayed gastric emptying, pelvic floor dysfunction, constipation, and SIBO as well. One cause of the gastrointestinal disorders is hypermobility of the bowels, which causes the bowels to fall into the pelvic space when you stand. This is called visceroptosis. This makes it difficult for the bowels and stomach to push forward, and as a result, SIBO is very common. There's no specific or genetic test for EDS and it is diagnosed by clinical history and physical examination. Patients with EDS require a multidisciplinary team of internists, rheumatologists, gastroenterologists, physiotherapists, and nutritionists for optimal care. If you have SIBO and you don't respond to treatment, it's important to rule out EDS.

Intra-abdominal adhesions from previous surgery or abdominal trauma can mechanically block the bowel and lead to bloating and abdominal distention. We see intra-abdominal adhesions among our IBS patients, but the relationship between these adhesions and positive breath tests has not been established in the scientific literature, despite our knowledge that there is a connection.

In a patient with **endometriosis**, the lining of the uterus can find its way into the abdominal cavity and grow on the bowel, bladder, or pelvic wall. During the menstrual cycle, the endometrial tissue can expand and cause abdominal pain and distention, symptoms that are often attributed to IBS. Classically, the abdominal pain tends to coincide with the menstrual cycle. Women who have irregular periods often have confusing abdominal symptoms.

Scleroderma is an autoimmune disease linked to IBS and anti-vinculin antibodies. In fact, the highest anti-vinculin antibodies we see are in scleroderma patients. We don't know why, but it's the only other disease (besides IBS) that displays these antibodies. The gastrointestinal form of scleroderma causes the lining of the tissues in the intestine to thicken. SIBO symptoms are common because the gut is stiff and doesn't move well, leading to the buildup of bacterial overgrowth.

Summary

This is not an exhaustive list of the diseases that cause bloating or diarrhea. For example, infections with *Clostridioides difficile* or giardia can also cause diarrhea. The workup for diarrhea and bloating can be quite extensive. The diseases and disorders we've described can be enigmas in the gastrointestinal clinic and chalked up to SIBO or misrepresented as SIBO, but there may be more going on than what meets the eye.

If you have one of these diseases, it doesn't mean that you don't have SIBO. They can overlap and cause bacterial overgrowth. Both IBS and SIBO are extraordinarily common, so you're more likely to have those conditions rather than any of the above-mentioned rarer diseases.

If your breath and antibody tests are positive, we hope that you can resolve your symptoms by following the path we've outlined in this book. We believe that you *can* manage the functional symptoms of IBS.

In the next chapter, we describe the current state of evidence with probiotics, prebiotics. and fecal transplantation.

CHAPTER 10

Probiotics, Prebiotics, and Fecal Transplantation

No discussion of the relationship between bacterial overgrowth and IBS can avoid mentioning so-called "good" bacteria, also known as probiotics, and their potential benefits as an aid against so-called "bad" bacteria.

Many of our patients ask us about "good" and "bad" bacteria, and we tell them that there's really is no such thing as "good" and "bad" native bacteria in the gastrointestinal tract. Actually, when it comes to the gastrointestinal tract, the concept of "good" bacteria is a misnomer. Very few of the thousands of strains of bacteria in the gastrointestinal tract are in fact "good" or "bad."

The concept of "good" bacteria has been largely promoted by the companies that manufacture probiotics. Even the first three letters "pro" have a positive flavor. Probiotics may be useful at times, and we've had patients tell us that their IBS symptoms improved when they used probiotics. We can't argue with that, however, IBS, as well as the health of the gastrointestinal tract in general, is far too complex to support a simple claim that certain types of bacteria will solve the problem.

IBS patients are often advised to have a stool sample cultured or analyzed to ascertain whether or not they have adequate amounts of "good" bacteria, such as lactobacillus and bifidobacteria. If the levels of these bacteria are found to be low, doctors may suggest they replenish them with probiotic supplements. Some data suggests that IBS patients have lower lactobacillus numbers in their stool, especially if they have diarrhea-predominant IBS. We now know that probiotic supplementation has shown little long-term benefit for IBS patients.

Other IBS patients are advised to take prebiotics, which serve as food for probiotics, or a combination of probiotics and prebiotics called synbiotics. This chapter will address these supplements, as well as *fecal microbiota transplantation*, also known as fecal transplant or stool transplant, and the potential for a statin-based treatment of IBS with constipation. All of these modalities are in the IBS therapy pipeline.

Probiotics Frenzy

The notion that probiotic supplements would benefit IBS patients began in the 1980s, and the probiotics frenzy continued through the 2000s. The two most popular forms of probiotics are *Lactobacillus acidophilus* and *Bifidobacterium bifidum*. Some tests of stool samples show lesser amounts of lactobacillus and bifidobacterium in IBS patients as compared with healthy people. Probiotic proponents have seized on these findings as evidence that IBS and other gastrointestinal disorders, including bacterial overgrowth, are due in part to deficiencies in one or both of these two types of bacteria. The problem with this notion is that most IBS patients have already figured out that drinking milk and eating dairy leads to symptoms (especially if they have SIBO). Milk and other dairy products are, in essence, a prebiotic to feed and increase *Lactobacillus acidophilus* in the gut. Take any group of people and starve them of dairy and they're likely to show a lack of *Lactobacillus acidophilus* in their bowels. The deficiency of *Lactobacillus acidophilus* in IBS patients may have been an artifact of a self-imposed dairy-free diet.

If the lack of these two bacteria was *the* problem that caused IBS, then probiotic supplements should reverse symptoms. In fact, a number of controlled studies show limited benefits from probiotics, and one recent double-blind study found that there were no measurable improvements among IBS patients who were given *Lactobacillus acidophilus*. There was, however, some improvement in IBS symptoms among patients who were given *Bifibacterium bifidum*. Any reduction in symptoms is a good outcome, but it's not the same as eliminating IBS altogether. At this time, scientific studies have not shown that probiotics eliminate IBS.

Some studies indicate that probiotic supplements may not always be safe. There have been case reports of negative side effects among children who were given large doses of *Lactobacillus acidophilus* to help treat their diarrhea. In one case, a child developed endocarditis (infection of the heart valve) as a result of over-consumption of *Lactobacillus acidophilus*. There have also been reported cases of blood infection in those who consumed too many probiotic supplements. All that said, these reports are very rare.

The real question concerning bacteria is not whether they are truly "good" or "bad," but where in the body they are located and how they interact with the rest of the microbiome and host. As with real estate, the most important issue is location, location, location. If bacteria are where they're supposed to be and doing what they're supposed to do, that's good. But if bacteria migrate to the wrong place, they can create problems.

For example, it's perfectly normal to find some *E. coli* bacteria in the stool, but if these bacteria migrate into the bloodstream and get into the urine, they can cause a potentially dangerous urinary tract infection. As you know from what you've already read, bacteria that migrate and overpopulate the small intestine can create problems, as so often happens with SIBO.

There's no question that certain types of bacteria—such as *Lactobacillus acidophilus* and *Bifidobacterium bifidum*—can have beneficial effects on the health of the gastrointestinal tract if they're not overconsumed. One study in Europe showed that these two bacteria can increase the cleaning-wave activity of the small intestine, which may be beneficial in SIBO patients. With hundreds of different types of bacteria in the gastrointestinal tract, it's unlikely that one type of bacteria alone, or even a combination of bacteria, can compensate for the effects of all the other bacteria. The composition of the gut bacteria is a complex mixture. Altering one or two bacteria is unlikely to treat any gastrointestinal disease.

Probiotics Challenges

Interestingly, in many conditions, the reason a treatment doesn't appear to work is because there hasn't been much research in the area. In fact, in IBS, there are many randomized controlled trials of probiotics, but most studies show no statistically significant improvement in IBS symptoms with probiotics over placebo.

To address the lack of effect of probiotics in IBS, investigators have published what's called a meta-analysis (an analysis of numerous studies). This pools all the individual studies into one major study. One such meta-analysis appears to show some significance that might nudge probiotics to the positive side of improvement. While meta-analysis is a good technique to pull together underpowered studies, sometimes lumping data together is like putting all the apples together without sorting the rotten ones from the good ones. There is also publication bias to consider. Journals (and researchers) don't publish negative studies, especially if they're small. Another problem with the meta-analysis of probiotics is that it combined studies of the bacteria *Lactobacillus acidophilus*, *Bifidobacterium bifidum*, and *saccharomyces* and claimed they were equivalent, when in fact they're totally different microorganisms with unique effects. The bottom line: There is no definitive conclusion that probiotics are beneficial for IBS.

Another meta-analysis of probiotic use in SIBO found that probiotics may have some benefit. Again, most of the data that exists for probiotics in SIBO is negative, with the exception of this particular meta-analysis.

The premise of this book is that SIBO is due to a disproportionate quantity of bacteria in the gut. Is it sensible to add more bacteria to the gut if you already have too much due to poor motility? This notion doesn't make sense to us. We've taken more SIBO patients off probiotics than put them on probiotics. We don't see a rationale for using probiotics in SIBO.

Some researchers rationalize the use of probiotics in SIBO because of the other properties of bacteria. Bifidobacterium, for example, can promote emptying of the stomach and it has also showed anti-inflammatory effects in physiologic studies. It can move bacteria around in the gut, compete with other bacteria, and change the balance of gut bacteria. Bifidobacterium has some interesting properties, but it has not panned out in the real world.

The side effects of probiotics present another potential problem. There are so many probiotic formulations and doses that no one can possibly study all the combinations to assess potential dangers. A study published in *The Lancet* in 2013 by researchers in the United Kingdom included 3000 patients who took probiotics or a placebo after a course of antibiotics. These were not IBS or SIBO patients per se. The patients were followed for 12 weeks to see whether they developed a *Clostridium difficile* infection or antibiotic-induced diarrhea. The rates of infection and diarrhea were exactly the same with probiotics and placebo. The only difference between the two groups was that the probiotics caused more bloating and flatulence. The end result: the probiotics caused more complications and showed no preventive effects after antibiotics. To be fair, the researchers used a specific cocktail of bacteria, so it may not be correct to say the result is true for all probiotics.

The researchers in this trial made sure the probiotics in the capsules were alive. One problem with probiotic supplements in the real world is that these microorganisms may die on the pharmacy shelf. Multiple studies from South Africa, Canada, the US, and Europe have shown that up to half of probiotic supplements don't contain the right amount, the right strain, or the live probiotics listed on the label.

Probiotics may cause problems in immunocompromised patients who lack the ability to respond normally to an infection due to an impaired or weakened immune system. Studies show multiple complications among infants, including *Lactobacillus acidophilus* leakage into the blood. For adults with severe pancreatitis (a sudden inflammation of the pancreas that may be mild or life-threatening), probiotics as compared to placebo showed harm with more infections and death. This is a red flag for sick patients, who probably should not take probiotic supplements.

Returning to our analogy of a large microbiome city in the gut, the notion that adding a strain or two of bacteria into this complex network of bacteria and fungi will fix the problem is naïve. Two recent studies of thousands of patients in the *New England Journal of Medicine* showed that probiotics don't protect against viral gastroenteritis. The majority of large studies so far show that probiotics are not a positive influence on the gut.

To be clear, we haven't dismissed probiotics yet, but we need precise studies with probiotic supplements designed to provide exactly the right dose as an individualized, tailored treatment. If we find that a particular probiotic does what it is supposed to do clinically, we will suggest that our patients take it. Future studies may show that they do indeed have a place in the overall treatment of IBS and SIBO. At this point in time, however, they only appear to provide some symptom relief rather than a comprehensive solution.

Prebiotics

Prebiotics are usually composed of dietary fiber that is designed to feed the bacteria in your gut. Prebiotics are found in many high-fiber foods, including some fruits, vegetables, and whole grains. Because prebiotics occur naturally in many foods, you don't need to take prebiotic supplements.

Prebiotics, which are not living organisms, essentially promote the growth of "healthy" microorganisms. They attempt to provide a specific composition that promotes a bacterium of interest. However, many bacteria besides the one of interest can use this prebiotic for growth. If you have SIBO, taking a prebiotic may actually provide food for the bacteria you don't want to overgrow. We've also found that prebiotics cause more bloating in our patients.

The evidence supporting prebiotics supplements for IBS is still preliminary. It's difficult to do a before-and-after study of the effects of prebiotics by looking at the microbiome in a stool sample. We can detect changes in the stool when our patients take prebiotics, but we don't yet know what a good effect would look like.

Synbiotics

A combination of probiotics and prebiotics is called *synbiotics* because they form a synergy of both. The idea behind synbiotics is that adding prebiotics to a probiotic supplement can help ensure that the digestion-friendly microorganisms arrive in the gut alive and well.

Theoretically, this makes sense because you're taking bacteria packed with its own food to help it grow. But there's not a lot of data to show that synbiotics are effective in treating IBS. Synbiotics are even harder to study than either probiotics or prebiotics alone because they add an extra layer of complexity to the gut microbiome. You're looking at two variables (probiotics and prebiotics) combined in one pill. Furthermore, the FDA doesn't supervise probiotics or prebiotics, as they're considered food, not medication; that's why it's very difficult to stop probiotics that don't have active bacteria from getting on the market. The lack of regulation doesn't guarantee that the product you buy is actually a synbiotic, or that it's effective at all.

When our patients tell us they are taking probiotics, prebiotics, or synbiotics and they feel better, we don't stop them from taking them. However, we don't suggest our patients take these supplements because we don't feel there's enough scientific evidence to support their use. Patients may indeed feel better due to the placebo effect because they believe in the treatment. If you expect a pill to do something, your body's chemistry may lead you to feel that the pill is working. In certain conditions, including IBS, a placebo can produce results even when you know you're taking a placebo.

Fecal Transplant

A *fecal transplant* is the transplantation of feces from a healthy donor into another person to restore the balance of bacteria in the gut. You could say that fecal transplant is the ultimate probiotic designed to change the gut's microbiome. But unlike a probiotic, which introduces a few strains of bacteria into the gut, a fecal transplant introduces a complete microbiome from a "healthy" person into the gut of a sick person.

Fecal transplant works particularly well to treat *Clostridioides difficile* infection; in fact, the FDA has approved fecal transplantation for the treatment of recurrent *Clostridioides difficile*. Unlike probiotics, the FDA considers stool a medication. Fecal transplants have also been tried in inflammatory bowel disease and ulcerative colitis, with mixed results.

For IBS, fecal transplant may have a theoretical benefit, but it's in no way a miracle. In six randomized controlled trials of fecal transplant in IBS, one trial was positive, one was barely positive, one was neutral, one was negative, and two were strongly negative (the placebo worked better than the transplant).

The two largest, most robust trials were conducted in Denmark and the US and they were both negative. These trials used a capsule that contained a fecal sample from a healthy person. In the Danish study, placebo capsules (which did not contain a healthy person's fecal sample) were statistically superior to fecal transplant in terms of improving IBS symptoms.

Interestingly, when the researchers checked the stool microbiome of the IBS patients after fecal transplantation, they found it looked like the healthy donor's microbiome, whereas the placebo pills had no effect on the stool microbiome. The transplant made the patients' stool look like a normal person's stool, but the IBS patients still had symptoms. This tells us that the source of IBS symptoms is in the small intestine, not the colon. Stool testing doesn't check the microbiome of the small intestine, and therefore doesn't show what the microbiome looks like in the small intestine and how it should be changed.

The US study showed similar results. An interim analysis of this randomized controlled trial found the placebo pills were superior to fecal transplantation, and the trial was stopped to avoid potential harm to patients.

Another study by Harvard researchers examined treating IBS with antibiotics, followed by a fecal transplant. The IBS patients received either antibiotics (rifaximin or metronidazole) or placebo pills, followed by a fecal transplant. The results showed no difference in IBS symptoms whether the patients took an antibiotic or placebo before fecal transplant, again adding to the disappointing results of fecal transplant in IBS.

Fecal transplantation can also carry potentially serious consequences. In the short-term, fecal transplantation can cause bloating and abdominal distention and diarrhea. We're still learning about the long-term consequences. In 2019, the FDA reported two deaths from multidrug-resistant bacteria during fecal transplantation in two immunocompromised patients. Recent US studies in fecal transplantation are now being reevaluated to look for multidrug-resistant bacteria.

In addition, the Harvard researchers saw some fecal transplant patients develop IBS-like symptoms from recurrent *Clostridioides difficile* infections. The researchers checked the donors' stool to try to explain these symptoms.

If the donor had SIBO, the fecal transplant recipient had a 50 percent chance of developing IBS after the transplant. If the donor didn't have SIBO, the risk of IBS symptoms was only 15 percent. Such results show that donor stool should not come from someone with SIBO, as chances are the SIBO will be passed to the recipient. This is difficult to explain, but of great interest to us.

In fact, we were the first doctors to report SIBO as a complication of fecal transplantation in a patient who had recurrent *Clostridioides difficile* infection. This patient received fecal transplantation and became extremely bloated with abdominal distention and constipation despite resolution of the *Clostridioides difficile* infection. We discovered that she had severe methane-predominant bacterial overgrowth, and when we treated her with multiple modalities, her symptoms improved. We discovered that this patient knew her fecal transplant donor, and we asked the donor to do a breath test. Lo and behold, the donor had a methane-positive breath test, too. The patient had received a transplant of donor stool to protect against *Clostridioides difficile*, but the sample also contained methane-producing archaea. The donor only suffered from mild constipation symptoms. This shows that one person (the donor) with normal motility can have mild symptoms, while another person (the IBS patient) with poor motility can have severe symptoms, even though they have exactly the same microbiome.

The ultimate goal of probiotics and prebiotics is to change the stool's microbiome. Researchers have tried to do this with fecal transplants and found it didn't work for patients with IBS. At the moment, we do not think an empiric fecal transplant is the best way to treat IBS or SIBO. Along with other researchers, we're working diligently to find out what determines the best response to fecal transplant, and what characteristics of donor stool and of the recipient's microbiome determine which patients may benefit the most from fecal transplantation.

Statin Therapy

Earlier in this book, we described the association between IBS with constipation and high levels of methane in breath tests, and the evidence that suggests that methane may slow down transit in the gastrointestinal tract.

We also noted that statins, specifically lovastatin, appear to decrease the generation of methane in stool samples. Lovastatin blocks methane production, but may not act as an antibiotic.

One of the issues we need to address in this research is a better understanding of the action mechanism of statins and how it relates to the growth of microorganisms that lead to methane production. We hope our research will lead to a treatment for IBS patients with constipation who need to reduce their intestinal methane production. Clinical studies that evaluate statins for the treatment of IBS with constipation have had mixed results, and further clinical trials are necessary. In addition, this research might lead to the development of economic methods to curb the production of the greenhouse gas methane, which could benefit all humankind.

Our final chapter aims to dispel many of the myths that continue to surround IBS.

CHAPTER 11

Myth Busting

I n this chapter, we address some myths about IBS and SIBO. This is not a comprehensive list of myths, but we include the top 10 questions we are asked, as well as other topics our patients are confused about. We covered some of this material earlier in the book, but the topics deserve to be reiterated.

Every IBS patient struggles with the emotions of living with IBS, and we don't dismiss anyone's feelings. We know you're suffering, and we've designed our protocol to help relieve symptoms, both physical and emotional.

Myth #1

SIBO is not a real medical condition.

This is false. Most gastroenterologists recognize the role of bacterial overgrowth in IBS; however, there are still some physicians who are unfamiliar with the emerging research that links bacterial overgrowth to IBS. Others dismiss the concept without taking the time to study the evidence. Today's physicians are inundated with medical information and may have a difficult time sifting through the large quantity of research to draw their own conclusions. They may become susceptible to the influence of traditional ideas about IBS, which do not include SIBO.

New concepts take years to be adopted by internists and gastro-enterologists, and even some highly advanced clinicians still don't recognize that IBS is not a woman's disease or simply caused by stress. In reality, we're all biased. We study gut microbes in IBS and to that extent we're highly focused on this area. But one should always remain open-minded to other possibilities.

If you see a physician for SIBO and they suggest you take a vacation or an antidepressant, this is 20-year-old advice that doesn't represent the current thinking about SIBO treatment. We're not saying a vacation doesn't help; we're saying that there's more to discuss and alternate ways to deal with SIBO. In this book, we've synthesized our protocol on how to treat IBS and SIBO based on multiple scientific studies we've published. Our ultimate goal is to prove that bacterial overgrowth causes many of the problems in IBS cases in double-blind studies. Importantly, other researchers have reproduced our findings with their own studies and clinical trials.

We aren't able to see every IBS patient in North America in our clinic. We wrote this book to empower patients and their family members and to educate physicians about SIBO. In 2021, most gastroenterologists in every corner of the country are well-versed in SIBO, particularly those at major medical centers. As a patient, you should evaluate whether or not your physician is helping you with your health problem. That includes asking yourself if the treatment provided to you is relieving your symptoms. If, after a reasonable period of time, you find you're not getting the care you deserve, you may need to look for other options.

Myth #2

Stomach acid can be replaced with oral supplementation.

This is false. The absence of cleaning waves is known to cause bacterial overgrowth. Another factor that can influence bacterial overgrowth is a lack of stomach acid. Undetected stomach abnormalities can lead to a lack of stomach acid production. For example, an autoimmune disease of the *parietal cells*—the epithelial cells that secrete hydrochloric acid in the stomach—can impair digestion of food. This disease is not common, so it can't be a common cause of SIBO.

Some health-care providers prescribe hydrochloric acid tablets for their SIBO patients to help with acid production, but the stomach produces two liters (about half a gallon) of acid each day. Taking a few tablets of hydrochloric acid doesn't make physiologic sense as SIBO treatment.

Furthermore, because lack of stomach acid is not a common cause of SIBO, it's unlikely that hydrochloric acid supplementation will alleviate the problem. In fact, supplementation could even be detrimental, because adding more acid to the gut may fuel more methane production (recall that methane-producing archeae use the hydrogen in acid to make methane), thus making constipation symptoms of SIBO even worse.

In a large study, we have shown that antacids do not increase the chance of SIBO, likely because antacids don't change the acidity of the small bowel, which is controlled by the pancreas. The main contributor of SIBO is the small bowel housekeeping wave, which is not affected by the acid produced in the stomach.

Myth #3

IBS is more common in women because they have a lower threshold for pain.

This is false. IBS is *not* a female disease, and has nothing to do with women being more sensitive to pain or more prone to anxiety. Yes, there are gender differences in IBS, depending on the symptoms. For those with extreme constipation, women outnumber men eight to one. For those with diarrhea, men outnumber women two to one. Gender has a role in IBS, but it is not to blame.

Women do have alterations in their IBS symptoms based on their menstrual cycle. Some women say their symptoms improve during menstruation and others say their symptoms worsen. Progesterone, one of the hormones involved in the menstrual cycle, has motility effects and can cause gut disturbances. We know that progesterone plays a role in IBS and menstruation, but we don't know exactly what that role is.

IBS after infectious gastroenteritis is also more common in women, but that's not surprising as most autoimmune disorders are more common in women and the presence of anti-vinculin autoantibodies is not an exception.

Myth #4

Restricted diets are safe in the long-term.

This is false. If you have IBS and you stop eating all food, your symptoms will improve dramatically. The bacteria wouldn't have food, but neither would you! When your gut doesn't work as hard, your symptoms dissipate, but a restricted diet is not a good long-term plan to control IBS. If you continue an overly restrictive diet for more than a few weeks, you may become deficient in macronutrients and micronutrients. The standard recommendation for more restricted diets is to reintroduce foods slowly within two to six weeks after starting the diet.

There is no one answer to the question of which foods to reintroduce first. This depends on the restricted diet you were on and what you were eating. The most important thing is to regain balance in your diet, which may require the help of a dietitian or nutritionist.

We also hear patients say, "I don't want to get IBS so I put myself on a low-FODMAP diet" or "I'm gluten sensitive and have put my children on a gluten-free diet to prevent them from getting celiac disease." There is no evidence that going on a restricted diet will protect you or your children from developing a gastrointestinal disorder.

Myth #5

Symptom alleviation with antidepressants, antipsychotics, narcotics, or behavioral therapy means IBS is all in your head.

This is false. One statement from IBS patients triggers the "all in your head" button with physicians: my IBS gets worse when I'm stressed. A more important question to ask yourself is, "Do I still have symptoms even when I'm not stressed?"

Stress can affect your bowel habits; for example, a problem at work, a serious exam, difficulties at home, and even a happy event like getting married or receiving a promotion can make your bowels behave differently, perhaps making underlying IBS symptoms worse. Under stressful circumstances, the colon will be more active and the cleaning waves may slow down or stop.

Stress is not believed to cause IBS. Even when the stress stops, the symptoms of IBS don't go away. We have patients who tell us that even when they go on vacation to a relaxing place, they still suffer from IBS symptoms. As we've mentioned, we eat, sleep, and exercise differently when we're under stress. All these changes can lead to a significant change in bowel pattern.

The concept of using antidepressants to treat IBS reinforces the notion that IBS is a psychological disorder. The therapies mentioned above (like antidepressants) are used for their specific side effects. For example, tricyclic antidepressants are anticholinergic—they dry mucous membranes and can cause constipation, but as a result help diarrhea. Antidepressants and narcotics like morphine cause constipation, and therefore may help in IBS with diarrhea. But that doesn't make them good treatments for IBS because they may be covering up the symptoms rather than determining the root cause.

We wrote a paper evaluating the harm of certain drugs in IBS, using the metric "number needed to harm." Drugs like tricyclics don't do well using this metric. In this study, 2.3 people would benefit from tricyclic antidepressants for IBS before one person had to stop the drug due to a side effect or harm. Contrast that to rifaximin, where 846 people would get better before another person might experience a side effect and have to stop the drug. We've published a paper that systematically summarizes the shortcomings of trials that assessed antidepressants in IBS patients. These trials usually have small sample sizes with variable design. More importantly, a significant proportion of these trials didn't properly report the adverse events and side effects.

Myth #6

If I have inflammatory bowel disease (IBD) or celiac disease, then I can't have IBS.

This is false. A great many patients with IBD or celiac disease also have bacterial overgrowth. The gut is affected by both of these diseases, which often leads to SIBO. We've shown that if you have IBD under control with anti-inflammatory drugs and still have IBS symptoms, you have a 57 percent chance of bacterial overgrowth. With celiac disease, those who have a partial response to a gluten-free diet commonly have SIBO, and they respond to SIBO treatments with antibiotics.

If you've been successfully treated for IBD or celiac disease and you still have symptoms, you may have SIBO as well. They are not mutually exclusive. Think of it this way: more than 10 percent of the US population has IBS/SIBO, so you could have any disease—lupus, osteoarthritis, or diabetes—and also have IBS/SIBO.

Myth #7

Federal research funding directly correlates with disease burden.

This is false. The US federal government has funded annually approximately one-quarter of a billion dollars for research into IBD, which affects 1.2 million Americans. In contrast, IBS researchers received $10 million to $15 million for a disease that affects 40 million Americans. In other words, IBS is funded at a rate that's 20 times less than IBD even though it's a more common disease and very problematic.

You may also notice the difference in advertising. For every IBS commercial you see on TV, there are 10 others for ulcerative colitis or Crohn's disease. More research means many more treatments for IBD compared to IBS. We're not implying that IBD or any other disease's funding should be diverted to IBS; however, we strongly believe that federal funding for IBS research must be dramatically increased.

Myth #8

IBS is a disease of developed countries.

This is false. IBS may appear to be a disease of the affluent in the US, but it's quite prevalent in both developed and undeveloped countries. The highest rates of IBS are found in Africa, Mexico, and Pakistan, where upwards of 40 percent of the population have IBS. Extreme forms of IBS and SIBO affect thousands of malnourished African children at a young age.

IBS is a global disease, with a prevalence of 11.2 percent worldwide. As the world becomes a global village with world travel, you're more likely to be exposed to different pathogens. The bottom line is that IBS can affect anyone, anywhere and in any country. It's a global problem.

Myth #9

Exercise makes IBS better.

This is true. Exercise increases blood flow to all organs, improves motility of the gut, and helps regulate bowel movements. Extreme exercise may be unfavorable to the gut due to a reduction of oxygen to the gut, but routine exercise is good for IBS patients. Studies of IBS patients show exercise assists in maintaining regular bowel habits. Exercise has the added benefit of releasing stress and, of course, provides many other health benefits.

Myth #10

IBS is contagious and hereditary.

This is false. The majority of IBS cases are caused by the connection to food poisoning and the associated poor motility. It is not contagious. Yes, you can transfer elements of your microbiome to another person by eating the same meals all the time, but that person won't get sick if they have normal gut motility.

More data suggests that your microbiome can look like your partner's microbiome, and even your dog can contribute to microbiome sharing by licking both partners. If one partner has IBS, it doesn't mean the other one will, and you can't transfer IBS to your partner through sexual intercourse. What you eat drives the composition of the microbiome. It's an environmental, not genetic, factor that matters.

In terms of bacterial overgrowth in IBS, once the food poisoning has done its damage, the resulting bacterial overgrowth itself is not contagious. You can't give it to someone else. That said, there are two instances of a genetic predisposition for IBS. If a parent has IBS with constipation and colonizes methane-producing organisms in the gut, their children may be more likely to have methane-producing organisms, which may lead to potential IBS symptoms when the children become adults.

A two-step process also hints at another predisposition for IBS. Only 11 percent of adults who have been infected with *Campylobacter* and have food poisoning develop IBS/SIBO. What creates the underlying risk that these adults are more likely to develop IBS/SIBO? If a mother has food poisoning, she may pass the inherent risk for IBS/SIBO to a child. Geneticists are working out the details of how this susceptibility may occur. It will, however, be difficult to prove that IBS is genetic because we can't eliminate other factors shared by family members that affect the microbiome.

In the same vein, celiac disease has genetic components. Nearly one-third of the general population carry the genes for celiac disease, but only one percent of them have celiac disease.

Conclusion

IBS has been stigmatized for many years. Patients are tired of hearing that it is "all in your head" and that they need to learn to "live with it." Numerous research studies show that IBS is *not* a psychological problem. We now know more about this disease and how the effects of the microbiome and imbalance of its microorganisms relate to IBS and SIBO.

We hope that the information in this book has convinced you that IBS is not "in your head." One of our main goals is to treat the disease as a gastrointestinal disorder. Now we know that food poisoning causes IBS and affects gut motility. We have hard, objective data on abnormalities in the gut caused by anti-vinculin in the setting of food poisoning, and abnormalities of the gut microbiome that lead to SIBO. These are not in your head. They are happening in your gut.

We now have a standardized method to diagnose bacterial overgrowth with breath testing and IBS with a blood test. Through our protocol, we've targeted multiple aspects of SIBO treatment, including diet, modification of the microbiome, and medical treatments. Low-fermentation eating was designed specifically to deal with SIBO. Over the past dozen or so years, we've used our experience with thousands of patients to design this way of eating. We now have a good handle on how to manage IBS and SIBO patients.

We're not finished! At any given time we have more than a dozen simultaneous research projects to further decipher this disease. We have more to come about how to modify your diet and how specifically to improve your microbiome and the body's interactions with the microbiome. Our research includes studying more specific gases that are involved in bacterial overgrowth, such as hydrogen sulfide; development of a new product for methane-predominant bacterial overgrowth; a non-antibiotic method to treat imbalances in the gut microbiome; and projects to suppress anti-vinculin production to eliminate antibodies from the blood. We've also invented devices to better draw samples from the bowels and have begun accumulating the largest database of the small intestine microbiome, not only with gastrointestinal disorders, but also with those involving neurologic, rheumatologic, and endocrine disorders. The end result of this research means that more help is coming.

Knowledge is empowerment. After reading this book, you know which interventions help relieve symptoms, which foods to eat to lessen the likelihood of symptoms, and what to do to avoid another bout of food poisoning. We hope this book gives you a better idea of what's true and what's not true in the IBS world. If you've read this entire book, you may know more about SIBO and IBS than many physicians do because it's hard for them to keep up with all diseases. This book can help you, as well as your doctor, improve your health.

If family members of IBS or SIBO patients also read this book, they'll begin to understand what you're going through. IBS is an invisible illness with no visible manifestations, but it's time for IBS to be recognized as a legitimate gastrointestinal disorder that can benefit from new theories and treatment strategies.

Low-Fermentation Eating Guide

SWEETENERS

FOOD TO CHOOSE (IN MODERATION)

Aspartame
(Equal or NutraSweet)

Glucose

Honey
(in small amounts)

Maple syrup

Sucrose
(table sugar)

FOOD TO AVOID (AS THEY'LL FEED BACTERIA)

High-fructose corn syrup

Inulin
(fiber food additive)

Lactitol
(sugar alcohol)

Lactose
(in dairy)

Maltitol/Mannitol
(sugar alcohols)

Sorbitol
(sugar alcohol)

Stevia

Sucralose
(Splenda)

Xylitol
(sugar alcohol)

CARBOHYDRATES

FOOD TO CHOOSE

Bagel, one half
(rye, sourdough, or plain)

Bread crumbs

Cereal, refined
(Rice Krispies, Original Special K,
cornflakes)

Cream of wheat

Dumpling wrappers

French bread

Gluten-free pasta made from
white rice, corn, or almond flour
(avoid those made
with brown rice or quinoa)

Gnocchi

Hemp seeds

Italian bread

Panko

Pasta

Phyllo dough

Popchips

Popcorn

Potato bread

Rice
(white, sushi, paella, jasmine)

Rice cakes
(made from white rice only)

Rye bread and crackers

Sourdough bread

Tortilla (corn or flour)

White or wheat bread
and crackers

Tip: Choose simple, easy-to-digest foods. Avoid high-fiber foods.

FOOD TO AVOID (AS THEY'LL FEED BACTERIA)

Beans and legumes

Bran

Brown rice

Multigrain bread

Oatmeal

Whole wheat bread and cereals

Whole wheat pasta

VEGETABLES

FOOD TO CHOOSE

Avocado

Beets

Capers

Caper berries

Carrots

Celeriac

Celery

Corn

Cucumber

Eggplant

Endive

English peas

Fennel root

Garlic
(small amount; cooked)

Green beans

Greens
(arugula, kale, spinach)

Horseradish

Jicama

Leek

Lettuce
(butter, romaine;
monitor carefully for symptoms)

Mushrooms

Olives

Onion
(small amount)

Parsnip

Peppers
(bell, chili)

Potato

Pumpkin

Radicchio

Rhubarb

Rutabaga

Scallion
(green part only)

Seaweed
(all types)

Shallot
(small amount; cooked)

Spinach

Squash
(summer, winter)

Sweet potato

Tomatillo

Tomato

Turnip

Water chestnut

Yam

Yucca

Zucchini

Tip: Keep salads to a small side salad only.

VEGETABLES (CONTINUED)

FOOD TO AVOID (AS THEY'LL FEED BACTERIA)

Artichoke

Asparagus

Beans and legumes

Broccoli

Brussels sprouts

Cabbage

Cauliflower

Edamame

Leafy vegetables
(although we think bacteria dislike spinach, kale, and arugula)

Pea pods

FRUITS

FOOD TO CHOOSE

Apricot, fresh

Avocado

Berries
(blackberries, blueberries, boysenberries, raspberries, strawberries)

Cherries

Citrus fruits
(orange, tangerine, grapefruit, lemon, lime)

Cranberries

Dragon fruit

Grapes

Guava

Kiwi

Mango

Melon, ½ cup
(cantaloupe, honeydew, watermelon)

Nectarine

Papaya

Passion fruit

Peach

Persimmon

Pineapple

Plum

Pomegranate

Tamarillo

FOOD TO AVOID (AS THEY'LL FEED BACTERIA)

Apple

Apricot, dried

Banana

Date

Dried fruits

Fig

Fruit-juice concentrates

Pear

Prune

PROTEINS

FOOD TO CHOOSE

Bacon
(without nitrates and
high-fructose corn syrup)

Beef

Eggs

Fish

Game

Lamb

Organ meats

Pork

Poultry

Seafood

Tips: Plain meats are fine, but be aware of how they are prepared. For example, they may be prepared in butter. Deli meats without starchy fillers are fine, but should be kept to a minimum. Watch for steak that is marinated when dining out. Also, most fine steak houses use a "butter finish," which makes the steak shine and taste richer. Ask for no finish.

FOOD TO AVOID (AS THEY'LL FEED BACTERIA)

Beans
(kidney, garbanzo
[chickpeas], lupini, pinto)

Breaded or
processed meats

Hummus
(made with chickpeas)

Lentils

Marinated steak
(steak house marinades
have high-fructose
corn syrup)

Tofu and soy products

Tip: Note that at Indian restaurants chickpea flour is used as gravy thickening and to make breads such as papadam. Ask your waiter.

DAIRY

FOOD TO CHOOSE

Butter
(small amount)

Cheese
(Asiago, Parmesan, cheddar,
Manchego, Gruyère)

Ghee

Lactose-free cottage cheese

Lactose-free milk
(almond milk, oat milk, pea milk)

Milk alternatives:

Almond milk

Coconut milk/cream

Hemp milk

Lactaid milk

Oat milk

Rice milk

DAIRY (CONTINUED)

FOOD TO AVOID (AS THEY'LL FEED BACTERIA)

Cheese not
mentioned above

Milk

Soy milk

Yogurt

Tip: Lactose-free yogurt and lactose-free sour cream are not recommended due to their live cultures. If you've been symptom-free for three months, you can have these occasionally.

FATS

FOOD TO CHOOSE

Butter in small amounts

Nut butter
(all natural, no additives)

Nuts
(almonds, cashews, chestnuts, coconut, hazelnuts, macadamia nuts, peanuts, pecans, pine nuts, pistachios, walnuts)

Oils
(avocado, canola, coconut, grapeseed, olive, sesame, sunflower, vegetable)

Seeds
(pumpkin seeds, sunflower seeds)

BAKED GOODS/SWEETS

FOOD TO CHOOSE

Active dry yeast

Agar flakes

All-purpose flour

Almond flour

Baking powder

Baking soda

Bittersweet chocolate

Cocoa powder

Corn flour

Cream of tartar

Dark chocolate

Instant coffee/espresso granules

Orange blossom water

Semisweet chocolate

Sorbet
(one scoop maximum)

Sugar
(cane, turbinado, caster)

Vanilla extract

Vanilla powder

CONDIMENTS

FOOD TO CHOOSE

Agave

Barbecue sauce without
high-fructose corn syrup
(FODY, Tessemae's)

Chile paste

Coconut aminos

Cornichons

Fish sauce

Gochujang

Honey
(in small amounts)

Jam made
from approved fruits

Ketchup without
high-fructose corn syrup
(Simply Heinz, Sir Kensington's,
Annie's Organic, Woodstock
Organic, Primal Kitchen)

Kuzu

Lord Sandy's Vegetarian
Worcestershire Sauce

Mayonnaise

Mustard with
allowed ingredients

Pickled ginger

Pomegranate molasses

Soy sauce

Sriracha

Tomato and pasta sauce with
allowed ingredients and
no additives
(Rao's Sensitive Marinara Sauce
for those who can't tolerate
onion or garlic)

Tomato paste

Vinegar
(pure, without additives)

FOOD TO AVOID (AS THEY'LL FEED BACTERIA)

Barbecue sauce with
high-fructose corn syrup

Ketchup with
high-fructose corn syrup

Plum sauce

Relish

Sweet and sour sauce

BEVERAGES

FOOD TO CHOOSE

Broth

Coffee

Juice of approved
fruits and vegetables
(small portions)

Seltzer or carbonated
beverages without
high-fructose corn syrup

Tea

Water

FOOD TO AVOID (AS THEY'LL FEED BACTERIA)

Drinks with
high-fructose corn syrup

Soda

ALCOHOL

FOOD TO CHOOSE

Beer
(low hops)

Bourbon

Brandy

Champagne

Gin

Grappa

Port

Rum

Sake

Sherry

Tequila

Vermouth

Vodka

Whiskey/Scotch

Wine
(red and white varieties)

Tip: Avoid sweetened mixers, which are high in sugar and may contain
high-fructose corn syrup.

Glossary

5-HT4 serotonin agonist A medication that activates 5-HT4 serotonin receptors (e.g., prucalopride) in the gut

Alpha-synuclein A protein that regulates nerve function and is involved in pathogenesis of Parkinson's disease

Anti-CdtB antibody An antibody with a cytolethal distending toxin-positive bacteria that develops after food poisoning

Anticholinergics Drugs that block the parasympathetic nervous system

Antihistamines Drugs that block the action of histamine to help with allergies

Anti-vinculin antibody An antibody that affects the function of the digestive system, commonly detected in post-infectious IBS

Antroduodenal manometry An advanced test that measures the contractions of the stomach and small bowel

Appendix A small tube-like pouch that connects to the cecum and can harbor bacteria and archaea

Archaea Resilient single-cell microorganisms found in the gut with various functions, such as methane production. They are among the oldest forms of life on earth.

Bacteroidetes A common group of bacteria with various functions that are abundant in the gut

Bile acid diarrhea (BAD) When excessive amounts of bile reach the colon, causing diarrhea. SIBO is one of the most common causes of BAD. Also known as bile acid malabsorption (BAM).

Bile acid malabsorption (BAM) When bile is not reabsorbed and excessive amounts reach the colon, causing diarrhea. SIBO is one of the most common causes of BAM. Also known as bile acid diarrhea (BAD).

Bile acids Specific acids that are synthesized in the liver and excreted into bile; they are very important in digestion of fat

Bile ducts Tubes in the liver that carry bile

Calcium channel blocker Drugs that block calcium channels, leading to relaxation of smooth muscles in various organs including the gut, heart, vessels, and bladder

Campylobacter jejuni A dangerous rod-like bacterium, it is the most common cause of food poisoning in North America

Candida A common fungus that can cause various diseases in humans including thrush, small intestinal fungal overgrowth, and candida vaginitis

Chyme A mixture of partially-digested food and stomach acid/enzymes that enter the small bowel from the stomach

Clostridioides difficile (C. difficile) An opportunistic bacterium that can cause inflammation of the colon. It commonly occurs after a course of antibiotics, especially in hospitals.

Collagenous colitis A type of colon inflammation that causes painless diarrhea. The inflammation can only be seen if the colon is biopsied during colonoscopy.

Colon The large intestine that connects to the small bowel at one end and the anus at the other; it contains and packages stool

Constipation IBS A type of IBS in which the predominant stool form is hard and lumpy

Crohn's disease A chronic inflammatory bowel disease that can involve any part of the gut, but it is most commonly found in the small bowel and colon

Disaccharides Sugars that derive from joining two monosaccharides; examples are lactose and sucrose (table sugar)

Duodenum The beginning of the small bowel in which pancreatic secretions and bile enter the intestine

Dyssynergic defecation Discoordination of the anal sphincter and abdominal muscles that makes it difficult to pass stool out; it can be a cause of constipation

Ehlers-Danlos Syndrome (EDS) A group of connective tissue diseases with various presentations. Hypermobile EDS can be associated with significant intestinal symptoms.

Endocannabinoid Compounds made by our body that are similar to compounds found in cannabis

Endometriosis A painful disease in which the tissue of the uterus lining finds its way out of the uterus and into the abdominal cavity

Escherichia coli (E. coli) A very common bacterium that is commonly found in the gut that can also cause various diseases, including sepsis, urinary infection, and traveler's diarrhea; one of the main bacteria that causes SIBO

Esophagus A muscular tube (swallowing pipe) that connects the mouth to the stomach

Fecal transplant The process of transferring stool from a donor to a recipient. Currently this is often used to treat recurrent *Clostridioides difficile* infection.

Firmicutes A common group of bacteria with various functions that are abundant in the gut

Fructan A highly fermentable form of sugar consisting of several connected fructose molecules

Fructose A monosaccharide found mostly in fruits

Gastrocolic reflex A reflex that activates movement of the large bowel when the stomach is filled with food; it explains why people sometimes have bowel movements after eating breakfast, for example

Glucose A monosaccharide that is easily absorbed in the gut

Gut microbiome Microbes and viruses, including bacteria, archaea, and microscopic eukaryotes, that live in the digestive tract

Gut motility A general term used to describe the movements of the gut that move the food through the digestive tract

Helicobacter pylori A spiral-shaped bacterium that survives in the stomach and is a major cause of stomach and duodenal ulcers

Hepatic encephalopathy Decreased brain function due to severe liver disease, which may be caused by the liver's inability to detoxify bacterial products that end up in the gut

Hirschsprung's disease A congenital disease of the large bowel in which there is a loss of nerve cells—mostly in the rectum—that causes severe constipation. Generally, this occurs in childhood.

Hydrogen An odorless gas that is exclusively produced by the gut microbiome and can be detected in the breath

Hydrogen sulfide A foul-smelling gas produced by bacteria and, to a lesser extent, by some human cells. Excessive hydrogen sulfide–producing bacteria can lead to diarrhea.

IBS-C A type of IBS in which the predominant stool form is hard and lumpy

IBS-D A type of IBS in which the predominant stool form is loose and watery

IBS-M A type of IBS in which the predominant stool form alternates between watery and hard at an irregular interval

Ileocecal valve A valve between the small bowel and large bowel; it prevents the contents of the large bowel from returning back into the small bowel

Ileum The last part of the small bowel that connects to the large bowel

Inflammatory bowel disease (IBD) Chronic recurrent inflammatory diseases of the bowel, generally presenting with ulceration of the bowel. The two main types are Crohn's disease and ulcerative colitis.

Intra-abdominal adhesions Formation of scar tissue within the abdomen that can fuse various organs and affect their function. It can cause SIBO when it narrows the small intestine and impairs good flow.

Inulin A type of fructan commonly added to foods, it can cause bloating in SIBO and IBS patients

Jejunum The middle part of the small bowel where the majority of nutrient absorption occurs

Klebsiella A rod-shaped bacterium that can cause various infectious diseases

Lactose A natural sugar found in dairy products consisting of two attached monosaccharides: galactose and glucose

Lactose intolerance It is defined as having symptoms of bloating and/or diarrhea after ingesting lactose-containing food (dairy products); it can be congenital or acquired (usually by food poisoning), due to loss of lactase (the enzyme that breaks down lactose). It can also be due to SIBO.

Lactulose A synthetic sugar that is not absorbable by humans but is fermentable by bacteria, which makes it ideal for breath testing for diagnosis of SIBO

Liver A large, solid organ in the abdomen that is in charge of detoxification, bile production, sugar storage, and various other functions

L-glutamine An essential amino acid that is integral to the health of the mucosal lining of the gut

Low-fermentation eating A lifestyle plan that involves eating to reduce the bacterial fermentation of food and decrease gastro-intestinal symptoms

Low-FODMAP diet A restrictive diet used for treatment of IBS

Lymphocytic colitis A type of microscopic colitis that presents with painless diarrhea. It is caused by inflammation in the colon only seen by taking a biopsy of the colon during colonoscopy.

Mast cell activation syndrome A disease state in which mast cells are hypersensitized and react excessively to stimuli, leading to numerous symptoms involving multiple systems

Methane An odorless gas that is exclusively produced by the gut micro-biome and can be detected in the breath

Methanobrevibacter smithii (M. smithii) The major type of methane-producing microbe in humans

Methanogens Methane-producing microbes (archaea)

Microbiome A collection of the bacteria, archaea, fungi, and viruses in our body, such as the gut, skin, and vaginal microbiomes

Microbiome gut-brain axis The notion that the gut microbiome and its composition can affect the brain (such as in mood disorder)

Migrating motor complex (MMC) Rhythmic contractions of the small bowel that are integral in the balance of gut microbiome. The MMC is needed to prevent SIBO.

Mitochodrial disorders Mitochondria are the energy-producing engines of our cells; their dysfunction leads to rare disorders with serious complications

Monosaccharide The most basic form of sugar that is readily absorbable by the gut. Examples are glucose, fructose, and galactose.

Mu-receptor agonist Drugs that block the effect of narcotics/opioids

Non-constipation IBS A term used to combine IBS-D and IBS-M (the two most common types of IBS) with a significant diarrheal component

Paleo Diet A diet that typically consists of lean meats, fish, nuts, seeds, fruits, and vegetables

Pancreas A solid organ that produces bicarbonate and several digestive enzymes as well as important hormones such as insulin

Pancreatic insufficiency Insufficient production of digestive enzymes produced by the pancreas, which leads to maldigestion of various nutrients, especially fat

Peristaltic waves Snake-like movement of the gut that moves food through the digestive tract

Peyer's patches Dense collections of lymphocytes (specific immune cells) that are found along the lining of the small bowel

Post-infectious dyspepsia The sensation of indigestion that occurs after food poisoning

Post-infectious gastroparesis The slow emptying of the stomach that happens after food poisoning; it presents with pain and vomiting

Post-infectious Guillain-Barré syndrome A paralyzing neurologic disease that commonly occurs after an infection (e.g., *Campylobacter jejuni* food poisoning)

Post-infectious IBS A very common type of IBS that occurs after food poisoning

Prokinetic drugs Drugs that help with the propagating movements of the gut

Proteobacteria A major group of bacteria that includes a large variety of pathogenic microbes, such as *E. Coli, Campylobacter, Salmonella, Shigella,* and *Helicobacter*

Psychosomatic A psychological condition that leads to physical symptoms. IBS was misunderstood as a psychosomatic disease and treated as such for a long time.

Psyllium A soluble fiber extracted from the seeds of a specific plant (*Plantago ovata*)

Pyloric sphincter A muscular valve between the stomach and the duodenum (the first part of the small intestine)

Reactive arthritis An inflammatory disease of the joints that occurs after some types of intestinal infections (e.g., *Campylobacter jejuni* food poisoning)

Rectum The last part of the large bowel (colon) where it connects to the anus

Salmonella A common bacterium and major cause of bacterial food poisoning; eggs and poultry are the most common source

Scleroderma A connective tissue disease that tightens/stiffens the skin, joints, and even internal organs such as the lungs. It significantly affects gut motility and is commonly associated with SIBO.

Serotonin A major nerve-control molecule; it is believed that 95 percent of all the serotonin in the body is in the gut

Shigella A common bacterium, associated with bloody traveler's diarrhea

Small intestinal bacterial overgrowth (SIBO) Excessive growth of bacteria in the small bowel that leads to various symptoms, including bloating and change in bowel habits

Small intestinal fungal overgrowth (SIFO) Excessive growth of fungi/yeast in the small bowel causing various symptoms, including bloating and change in bowel habits

Specific Carbohydrate Diet A restrictive diet free of grains, starch, and processed foods

Tachyphylaxis A sudden drop in drug effects due to rapid development of drug tolerance

Vagus nerve The longest autonomic nerve in the body that has a major role in the function of the heart, lungs, and the digestive system. Vagus nerve injury can lead to various GI symptoms.

Villi Finger-like projections from the lining of the small bowel that absorb the nutrients; they dramatically increase the surface area of the gut to optimize absorption

Vinculin A cell protein involved in cell migration. There are various forms of vinculin, but one specific form is important for the cells controlling gut motility.

ABOUT THE AUTHORS

Mark Pimentel, MD, FRCP(C)

Mark Pimentel, MD, FRCP(C), is professor of medicine and gastroenterology at Geffen School of Medicine UCLA and associate professor of medicine at Cedars-Sinai, Los Angeles. He is also the executive director of the Medically Associated Science and Technology (MAST) Program at Cedars-Sinai. A pioneering expert in irritable bowel syndrome (IBS), Dr. Pimentel has had his work published in *The New England Journal of Medicine, Annals of Internal Medicine, American Journal of Physiology, The American Journal of Medicine, American Journal of Gastroenterology,* and *Digestive Diseases and Sciences,* among others. His research led to the first-ever blood tests for IBS, with ibs-smart©, the only licensed and patented serologic diagnostic for IBS. Pimentel has served as a principal investigator or co-investigator for numerous translational and clinical investigations of IBS and the relationship between gut flora composition and human disease. Dr. Pimentel is a diplomate of the American Board of Internal Medicine, a fellow of the Royal College of Physicians and Surgeons of Canada, and a member of the American Gastroenterological Association, the American College of Gastroenterology, and the American Neurogastroenterology and Motility Society.

Ali Rezaie, MD, MSc, FRCP(C)

Ali Rezaie, MD, MSc, FRCP(C), is the medical director of the GI Motility Program at Cedars-Sinai, Los Angeles, and the director of the GI Motility Fellowship Training Program. He is an associate professor at Cedars-Sinai and an associate clinical professor at UCLA. Dr. Rezaie also serves as the director of Bioinformatics and Biotechnology for the Medically Associated Science and Technology (MAST) Program at Cedars-Sinai. Apart from his training in internal medicine and gastroenterology, he has postdoctoral training in gastrointestinal motility disorders and also inflammatory bowel diseases (IBD) as well as a master's degree in epidemiology. Dr. Rezaie has published more than 100 peer-reviewed papers that have been cited over 7000 times. Rezaie has been awarded multiple grants from prestigious organizations including the Canadian Institutes of Health Research fellowship, the American College of Gastroenterology Research, and the Kenneth Rainin Foundation. He also serves as the associate editor of *Digestive Diseases and Sciences,* a peer-reviewed journal of gastroenterology and hepatology. His research focuses on microbiome, irritable bowel syndrome (IBS), small intestinal bacterial overgrowth (SIBO), medical device development, and internal UV therapy.